UCV

BLACKWELL

UNDERGROUND CLINICAL VIGNETTES

PATHOPHYSIOLOGY I: PULMONARY, OB/GYN, ENT, HEM/ONC, 4E

BLACKWELL

UNDERGROUND CLINICAL VIGNETTES

PATHOPHYSIOLOGY I: PULMONARY, OB/GYN, ENT, HEM/ONC, 4E

VIKAS BHUSHAN, MD
Series Editor
University of California, San Francisco, Class of 1991
Diagnostic Radiologist

VISHAL PALL, MD MPH
Series Editor
Internist and Preventive Medicine Specialist
Government Medical College, Chandigarh – Panjab University – India, Class of 1997
Graduate School of Biomedical Sciences at UTMB Galveston, MPH, Class of 2004

TAO LE, MD
University of California, San Francisco, Class of 1996

ALI ASGHAR GAMINI, MD
Shiraz University School of Medicine, Class of 1994
Assistant Professor of Microbiology and Immunology, St. Luke's University School of Medicine

BAHAR SEDARATI, MD
Shiraz University School of Medicine, Class of 1995
Associate Professor, Department of Pathology, St. Luke's University School of Medicine

HOANG NGUYEN, MD, MBA
Northwestern University, Class of 2001

VIPAL SONI, MD
UCLA School of Medicine, Class of 1999

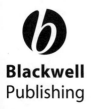

Blackwell
Publishing

Blackwell Publishing, Inc., 350 Main Street, Malden, Massachusetts 02148-5018, USA
Blackwell Publishing Ltd, 9600 Garsington Road, Oxford OX4 2DQ, UK
Blackwell Publishing Asia Pty Ltd, 550 Swanston Street, Carlton, Victoria 3053, Australia

05 06 07 08 5 4 3 2 1

ISBN-13: 978-1-4051-0414-2
ISBN-10: 1-4051-0414-7

Library of Congress Cataloging-in-Publication Data

Pathophysiology. Pulmonary system, Ob/Gyn, ENT, Hem/Onc / Vikas Bhushan . . . [et al.].— 4th ed.
    p. ; cm. — (Blackwell underground clinical vignettes)
    ISBN-13: 978-1-4051-0414-2 (pbk. : alk. paper)
    ISBN-10: 1-4051-0414-7 (pbk. : alk. paper)   1. Respiratory organs—Diseases—Case studies.
    [DNLM: 1. Respiratory Tract Diseases—Case Reports.   2. Respiratory Tract Diseases—Problems and Exercises.]   I. Bhushan, Vikas.   II. Bhushan, Vikas. Pathophysiology.   III. Series: Blackwell's underground clinical vignettes.

    RC711.P86 2005
    616.2'0076—dc22

                                                                                        2005003551

A catalogue record for this title is available from the British Library

Acquisitions: Nancy Anastasi Duffy
Development/Production: Jennifer Kowalewski
Cover and Interior design: Leslie Haimes
Typesetter: Graphicraft in Quarry Bay, Hong Kong
Printed and bound by Capital City Press in Berlin, VT

For further information on Blackwell Publishing, visit our website:
www.blackwellmedstudent.com

NOTICE

The indications and dosages of all drugs in this book have been recommended in the medical literature and conform to the practices of the general community. The medications described do not necessarily have specific approval by the Food and Drug Administration for use in the diseases and dosages for which they are recommended. The package insert for each drug should be consulted for use and dosage as approved by the FDA. Because standards for usage change, it is advisable to keep abreast of revised recommendations, particularly those concerning new drugs.

The authors of this volume have taken care that the information contained herein is accurate and compatible with the standards generally accepted at the time of publication. Nevertheless, it is difficult to ensure that all the information given is entirely accurate for all circumstances. The publisher and authors do not guarantee the contents of this book and disclaim any liability, loss, or damage incurred as a consequence, directly or indirectly, of the use and application of any of the contents of this volume.

The publisher's policy is to use permanent paper from mills that operate a sustainable forestry policy, and which has been manufactured from pulp processed using acid-free and elementary chlorine-free practices. Furthermore, the publisher ensures that the text paper and cover board used have met acceptable environmental accreditation standards.

CONTENTS

OB

ENT/OPHTALMOLOGY

HEM/ONC

CONTRIBUTORS

Sameer Sheth, PhD
David Geffen School of Medicine at UCLA, Class of 2005

Hui J Jenny Chen
David Geffen School of Medicine at UCLA, Class of 2005

Kaushik Mukherjee
David Geffen School of Medicine at UCLA, Class of 2005

Joseph Hastings
David Geffen School of Medicine at UCLA, Class of 2006
UCLA School of Public Health, MPH, Class of 2006

Kyong Un Chong
Joan C. Edwards School of Medicine, West Virginia, Class of 2005

Chad Silverberg
Philadelphia College of Osteopathic Medicine, Class of 2004
Resident in Internal Medicine, Cleveland Clinic Foundation
Radiology Resident, Christiana Hospital (From 2005)

Nazli Bolori, MD
St. Matthew's School of Medicine, Class of 2004
Clinical Researcher, Medstar Research Institute

Chris Buckle
University of Ottawa, Class of 2005

Mustaqeem A Siddiqui, MD
Aga Khan University Medical College, Class of 2002
Resident in Internal Medicine, Mayo Clinic, Rochester MN

Michael Kenneth Shindle, MD
Johns Hopkins University School of Medicine, Baltimore, MD, Class of 2004
Intern, Orthopedic Surgery, Hospital for Special Surgery, New York NY

Pourya M.Ghazi, MD
Senior Fellow, Department of Laboratory Medicine, University of Washington, Seattle

Robert Nason
University of Texas Medical Branch, Class of 2003

ACKNOWLEDGMENTS

Throughout the production of this book, we have had the support of many friends and colleagues. Special thanks to our support team including Andrea Fellows, Anastasia Anderson, Srishti Gupta, Anu Gupta, Mona Pall, Jonathan Kirsch and Chirag Amin. For prior contributions we thank Gianni Le Nguyen, Tarun Mathur, Alex Grimm, Sonia Santos and Elizabeth Sanders.

For submitting comments, corrections, editing, proofreading, and assistance across all of the vignette titles in all editions, we collectively thank:

Tara Adamovich, Carolyn Alexander, Kris Alden, Henry E. Aryan, Lynman Bacolor, Natalie Barteneva, Dean Bartholomew, Debashish Behera, Sumit Bhatia, Sanjay Bindra, Dave Brinton, Julianne Brown, Alexander Brownie, Tamara Callahan, David Canes, Bryan Casey, Aaron Caughey, Hebert Chen, Jonathan Cheng, Arnold Cheung, Arnold Chin, Simion Chiosea, Yoon Cho, Samuel Chung, Gretchen Conant, Vladimir Coric, Christopher Cosgrove, Ronald Cowan, Karekin R. Cunningham, A. Sean Dalley, Rama Dandamudi, Sunit Das, Ryan Armando Dave, John David, Emmanuel de la Cruz, Robert DeMello, Navneet Dhillon, Sharmila Dissanaike, David Donson, Adolf Etchegaray, Alea Eusebio, Jose M. Fierro, Priscilla A. Frase, David Frenz, Kristin Gaumer, Yohannes Gebreegziabher, Anil Gehi, Tony George, L.M. Gotanco, Parul Goyal, Alex Grimm, Rajeev Gupta, Ahmad Halim, Sue Hall, David Hasselbacher, Tamra Heimert, Michelle Higley, Dan Hoit, Eric Jackson, Tim Jackson, Sundar Jayaraman, Pei-Ni Jone, Aarchan Joshi, Rajni K. Jutla, Faiyaz Kapadi, Seth Karp, Aaron S. Kesselheim, Sana Khan, Andrew Pin-wei Ko, Francis Kong, Paul Konitzky, Warren S. Krackov, Benjamin H.S. Lau, Ann LaCasce, Connie Lee, Scott Lee, Guillermo Lehmann, Kevin Leung, Paul Levett, Warren Levinson, Eric Ley, Ken Lin, Pavel Lobanov, J. Mark Maddox, Aram Mardian, Samir Mehta, Gil Melmed, Joe Messina, Robert Mosca, Michael Murphy, Kristen Lem Mygdal, Vivek Nandkarni, Siva Naraynan, Carvell Nguyen, Linh Nguyen, Deanna Nobleza, Craig Nodurft, George Noumi, Darin T. Okuda, Adam L. Palance, Paul Pamphrus, Jinha Park, Sonny Patel, Ricardo Pietrobon, Riva L. Rahl, Aashita Randeria, Rachan Reddy, Beatriu Reig, Marilou Reyes, Jeremy Richmon, Tai Roe, Rick Roller, Rajiv Roy, Diego Ruiz, Anthony Russell, Sanjay Sahgal, Urmimala Sarkar, John Schilling, Isabell Schmitt, Daren Schuhmacher, Sonal Shah, Fadi Abu Shahin, Edie Shen, Justin Smith, John Stulak, Lillian Su, Julie Sundaram, Rita Suri, Seth Sweetser, Antonio Talayero, Merita Tan, Mark Tanaka, Eric Taylor, Jess Thompson, Indi Trehan, Raymond Turner, Okafo Uchenna, Eric Uyguanco, Richa Varma, John Wages, Alan Wang, Eunice Wang, Tisha Wang, Andy Weiss, Amy Williams, Brian Yang, Hany Zaky, Ashraf Zaman and David Zipf.

Please let us know if your name has been missed or misspelled and we will be happy to make the update in the next edition.

For generously contributing images to the entire Underground Clinical Vignette Step 1 series, we collectively thank the staff at Blackwell Publishing in Oxford, Boston, and Berlin as well as:

- Axford, J. Medicine. Osney Mead: Blackwell Science Ltd, 1996. Figures 2.14, 2.15, 2.16, 2.27, 2.28, 2.31, 2.35, 2.36, 2.38, 2.43, 2.65a, 2.65b, 2.65c, 2.103b, 2.105b, 3.20b, 3.21, 8.27, 8.27b, 8.77b, 8.77c, 10.81b, 10.96a, 12.28a, 14.6, 14.16, 14.50.

• Bannister B, Begg N, Gillespie S. Infectious Disease, 2nd Edition. Osney Mead: Blackwell Science Ltd, 2000. Figures 2.8, 3.4, 5.28, 18.10, W5.32, W5.6.

• Berg D. Advanced Clinical Skills and Physical Diagnosis. Blackwell Science Ltd., 1999. Figures 7.10, 7.12, 7.13, 7.2, 7.3, 7.7, 7.8, 7.9, 8.1, 8.2, 8.4, 8.5, 9.2, 10.2, 11.3, 11.5, 12.6.

• Cuschieri A, Hennessy TPJ, Greenhalgh RM, Rowley DA, Grace PA. Clinical Surgery. Osney Mead: Blackwell Science Ltd, 1996. Figures 13.19, 18.22, 18.33.

• Gillespie SH, Bamford K. Medical Microbiology and Infection at a Glance. Osney Mead.: Blackwell Science Ltd, 2000, Figures 20, 23.

• Ginsberg L. Lecture Notes on Neurology, 7th Edition. Osney Mead: Blackwell Science Ltd, 1999. Figures 12.3, 18.3, 18.3b.

• Elliott T, Hastings M, Desselberger U. Lecture Notes on Medical Microbiology, 3rd Edition. Osney Mead: Blackwell Science Ltd, 1997. Figures 2, 5, 7, 8, 9, 11, 12, 14, 15, 16, 17, 19, 20, 25, 26, 27, 29, 30, 34, 35, 52.

• Mehta AB, Hoffbrand AV. Haematology at a Glance. Osney Mead: Blackwell Science Ltd, 2000. Figures 22.1, 22.2, 22.3.

HOW TO USE THIS BOOK

This series was originally developed to address the increasing number of clinical vignette questions on medical examinations, including the USMLE Step 1 and Step 2.

Each UCV 1 book uses a series of approximately 100 "supra-prototypical" cases as a way to condense testable facts and associations. The clinical vignettes in this series are designed to give added emphasis to pathogenesis, epidemiology, management and complications. Although each case tends to present all the signs, symptoms, and diagnostic findings for a particular illness, patients generally will not present with such a "complete" picture either clinically or on a medical examination. Cases are not meant to simulate a potential real patient or an exam vignette. All the boldfaced "buzzwords" are for learning purposes and are not necessarily expected to be found in any one patient with the disease.

Definitions of selected important terms are placed within the vignettes in (small caps) in parentheses. Other parenthetical remarks often refer to the pathophysiology or mechanism of disease. The format should also help students learn to present cases succinctly during oral "bullet" presentations on clinical rotations. The cases are meant to serve as a condensed review, not as a primary reference. The information provided in this book has been prepared with a great deal of thought and careful research. This book should not, however, be considered as your sole source of information. Corrections, suggestions and submissions of new cases are encouraged and will be acknowledged and incorporated when appropriate in future editions.

We hope that you find the *Blackwell Underground Clinical Vignettes* series informative and useful. We welcome feedback and suggestions you have about this book, or any published by Blackwell Publishing.

Please e-mail us at medfeedback@bos.blackwellpublishing.com.

ABBREVIATIONS

ABGs	arterial blood gases
ABPA	allergic bronchopulmonary aspergillosis
ACA	anticardiolipin antibody
ACE	angiotensin-converting enzyme
ACL	anterior cruciate ligament
ACTH	adrenocorticotropic hormone
AD	adjustment disorder
ADA	adenosine deaminase
ADD	attention deficit disorder
ADH	antidiuretic hormone
ADHD	attention deficit hyperactivity disorder
ADP	adenosine diphosphate
AFO	ankle-foot orthosis
AFP	α-fetoprotein
AIDS	acquired immunodeficiency syndrome
ALL	acute lymphocytic leukemia
ALS	amyotrophic lateral sclerosis
ALT	alanine aminotransferase
AML	acute myelogenous leukemia
ANA	antinuclear antibody
Angio	angiography
AP	anteroposterior
APKD	adult polycystic kidney disease
aPTT	activated partial thromboplastin time
ARDS	adult respiratory distress syndrome
5-ASA	5-aminosalicylic acid
ASCA	antibodies to *Saccharomyces cerevisiae*
ASO	antistreptolysin O
AST	aspartate aminotransferase
ATLL	adult T-cell leukemia/lymphoma
ATPase	adenosine triphosphatase
AV	arteriovenous, atrioventricular
AZT	azidothymidine (zidovudine)
BAL	British antilewisite (dimercaprol)
BCG	bacille Calmette-Guérin
BE	barium enema
BP	blood pressure
BPH	benign prostatic hypertrophy
BUN	blood urea nitrogen
CABG	coronary artery bypass grafting
CAD	coronary artery disease
CaEDTA	calcium edetate
CALLA	common acute lymphoblastic leukemia antigen
cAMP	cyclic adenosine monophosphate
C-ANCA	cytoplasmic antineutrophil cytoplasmic antibody
CBC	complete blood count

CBD	common bile duct
CCU	cardiac care unit
CD	cluster of differentiation
2-CdA	2-chlorodeoxyadenosine
CEA	carcinoembryonic antigen
CFTR	cystic fibrosis transmembrane conductance regulator
cGMP	cyclic guanosine monophosphate
CHF	congestive heart failure
CK	creatine kinase
CK-MB	creatine kinase, MB fraction
CLL	chronic lymphocytic leukemia
CML	chronic myelogenous leukemia
CMV	cytomegalovirus
CN	cranial nerve
CNS	central nervous system
COPD	chronic obstructive pulmonary disease
COX	cyclooxygenase
CP	cerebellopontine
CPAP	continuous positive airway pressure
CPK	creatine phosphokinase
CPPD	calcium pyrophosphate dihydrate
CPR	cardiopulmonary resuscitation
CREST	calcinosis, Raynaud's phenomenon, esophageal involvement, sclerodactyly, telangiectasia (syndrome)
CRP	C-reactive protein
CSF	cerebrospinal fluid
CSOM	chronic suppurative otitis media
CT	cardiac transplant, computed tomography
CVA	cerebrovascular accident
CXR	chest x-ray
d4T	didehydrodeoxythymidine (stavudine)
DCS	decompression sickness
DDH	developmental dysplasia of the hip
ddI	dideoxyinosine (didanosine)
DES	diethylstilbestrol
DEXA	dual-energy x-ray absorptiometry
DHEAS	dehydroepiandrosterone sulfate
DIC	disseminated intravascular coagulation
DIF	direct immunofluorescence
DIP	distal interphalangeal (joint)
DKA	diabetic ketoacidosis
DL_{CO}	diffusing capacity of carbon monoxide
DMSA	2,3-dimercaptosuccinic acid
DNA	deoxyribonucleic acid
DNase	deoxyribonuclease
2,3-DPG	2,3-diphosphoglycerate

dsDNA	double-stranded DNA
DSM	Diagnostic and Statistical Manual
dsRNA	double-stranded RNA
DTP	diphtheria, tetanus, pertussis (vaccine)
DTPA	diethylenetriamine-penta-acetic acid
DTs	delirium tremens
DVT	deep venous thrombosis
EBV	Epstein-Barr virus
ECG	electrocardiography
Echo	echocardiography
ECM	erythema chronicum migrans
ECT	electroconvulsive therapy
EEG	electroencephalography
EF	ejection fraction, elongation factor
EGD	esophagogastroduodenoscopy
EHEC	enterohemorrhagic *E. coli*
EIA	enzyme immunoassay
ELISA	enzyme-linked immunosorbent assay
EM	electron microscopy
EMG	electromyography
ENT	ears, nose, and throat
EPVE	early prosthetic valve endocarditis
ER	emergency room
ERCP	endoscopic retrograde cholangiopancreatography
ERT	estrogen replacement therapy
ESR	erythrocyte sedimentation rate
ETEC	enterotoxigenic *E. coli*
EtOH	ethanol
FAP	familial adenomatous polyposis
FEV_1	forced expiratory volume in 1 second
FH	familial hypercholesterolemia
FNA	fine-needle aspiration
FSH	follicle-stimulating hormone
FTA-ABS	fluorescent treponemal antibody absorption test
FVC	forced vital capacity
G6PD	glucose-6-phosphate dehydrogenase
GABA	gamma-aminobutyric acid
GERD	gastroesophageal reflux disease
GFR	glomerular filtration rate
GGT	gamma-glutamyltransferase
GH	growth hormone
GI	gastrointestinal
GnRH	gonadotropin-releasing hormone
GU	genitourinary
GVHD	graft-versus-host disease
HAART	highly active antiretroviral therapy

HAV	hepatitis A virus
Hb	hemoglobin
HbA-1C	hemoglobin A-1C
HBsAg	hepatitis B surface antigen
HBV	hepatitis B virus
hCG	human chorionic gonadotropin
HCO_3	bicarbonate
Hct	hematocrit
HCV	hepatitis C virus
HDL	high-density lipoprotein
HDL-C	high-density lipoprotein-cholesterol
HEENT	head, eyes, ears, nose, and throat (exam)
HELLP	hemolysis, elevated LFTs, low platelets (syndrome)
HFMD	hand, foot, and mouth disease
HGPRT	hypoxanthine-guanine phosphoribosyltransferase
5-HIAA	5-hydroxyindoleacetic acid
HIDA	hepato-iminodiacetic acid (scan)
HIV	human immunodeficiency virus
HLA	human leukocyte antigen
HMG-CoA	hydroxymethylglutaryl-coenzyme A
HMP	hexose monophosphate
HPI	history of present illness
HPV	human papillomavirus
HR	heart rate
HRIG	human rabies immune globulin
HRS	hepatorenal syndrome
HRT	hormone replacement therapy
HSG	hysterosalpingography
HSV	herpes simplex virus
HTLV	human T-cell leukemia virus
HUS	hemolytic-uremic syndrome
HVA	homovanillic acid
ICP	intracranial pressure
ICU	intensive care unit
ID/CC	identification and chief complaint
IDDM	insulin-dependent diabetes mellitus
IFA	immunofluorescent antibody
Ig	immunoglobulin
IGF	insulin-like growth factor
IHSS	idiopathic hypertrophic subaortic stenosis
IM	intramuscular
IMA	inferior mesenteric artery
INH	isoniazid
INR	International Normalized Ratio
IP_3	inositol 1,4,5-triphosphate
IPF	idiopathic pulmonary fibrosis

ITP	idiopathic thrombocytopenic purpura
IUD	intrauterine device
IV	intravenous
IVC	inferior vena cava
IVIG	intravenous immunoglobulin
IVP	intravenous pyelography
JRA	juvenile rheumatoid arthritis
JVP	jugular venous pressure
KOH	potassium hydroxide
KUB	kidney, ureter, bladder
LCM	lymphocytic choriomeningitis
LDH	lactate dehydrogenase
LDL	low-density lipoprotein
LE	lupus erythematosus (cell)
LES	lower esophageal sphincter
LFTs	liver function tests
LH	luteinizing hormone
LMN	lower motor neuron
LP	lumbar puncture
LPVE	late prosthetic valve endocarditis
L/S	lecithin-sphingomyelin (ratio)
LSD	lysergic acid diethylamide
LT	labile toxin
LV	left ventricular
LVH	left ventricular hypertrophy
Lytes	electrolytes
Mammo	mammography
MAO	monoamine oxidase (inhibitor)
MCP	metacarpophalangeal (joint)
MCTD	mixed connective tissue disorder
MCV	mean corpuscular volume
MEN	multiple endocrine neoplasia
MI	myocardial infarction
MIBG	meta-iodobenzylguanidine (radioisotope)
MMR	measles, mumps, rubella (vaccine)
MPGN	membranoproliferative glomerulonephritis
MPS	mucopolysaccharide
MPTP	1-methyl-4-phenyl-tetrahydropyridine
MR	magnetic resonance (imaging)
mRNA	messenger ribonucleic acid
MRSA	methicillin-resistant *S. aureus*
MTP	metatarsophalangeal (joint)
NAD	nicotinamide adenine dinucleotide
NADP	nicotinamide adenine dinucleotide phosphate
NADPH	reduced nicotinamide adenine dinucleotide phosphate
NF	neurofibromatosis

NIDDM	non-insulin-dependent diabetes mellitus
NNRTI	non-nucleoside reverse transcriptase inhibitor
NO	nitric oxide
NPO	nil per os (nothing by mouth)
NSAID	nonsteroidal anti-inflammatory drug
Nuc	nuclear medicine
NYHA	New York Heart Association
OB	obstetric
OCD	obsessive-compulsive disorder
OCPs	oral contraceptive pills
OR	operating room
PA	posteroanterior
PABA	para-aminobenzoic acid
PAN	polyarteritis nodosa
P-ANCA	perinuclear antineutrophil cytoplasmic antibody
Pa_{O_2}	partial pressure of oxygen in arterial blood
PAS	periodic acid Schiff
PAT	paroxysmal atrial tachycardia
PBS	peripheral blood smear
P_{CO_2}	partial pressure of carbon dioxide
PCOM	posterior communicating (artery)
PCOS	polycystic ovarian syndrome
PCP	phencyclidine
PCR	polymerase chain reaction
PCT	porphyria cutanea tarda
PCTA	percutaneous coronary transluminal angioplasty
PCV	polycythemia vera
PDA	patent ductus arteriosus
PDGF	platelet-derived growth factor
PE	physical exam
PEFR	peak expiratory flow rate
PEG	polyethylene glycol
PEPCK	phosphoenolpyruvate carboxykinase
PET	positron emission tomography
PFTs	pulmonary function tests
PID	pelvic inflammatory disease
PIP	proximal interphalangeal (joint)
PKU	phenylketonuria
PMDD	premenstrual dysphoric disorder
PML	progressive multifocal leukoencephalopathy
PMN	polymorphonuclear (leukocyte)
PNET	primitive neuroectodermal tumor
PNH	paroxysmal nocturnal hemoglobinuria
P_{O_2}	partial pressure of oxygen
PPD	purified protein derivative (of tuberculosis)
PPH	primary postpartum hemorrhage

PRA	panel reactive antibody
PROM	premature rupture of membranes
PSA	prostate-specific antigen
PSS	progressive systemic sclerosis
PT	prothrombin time
PTH	parathyroid hormone
PTSD	post-traumatic stress disorder
PTT	partial thromboplastin time
PUVA	psoralen ultraviolet A
PVC	premature ventricular contraction
RA	rheumatoid arthritis
RAIU	radioactive iodine uptake
RAST	radioallergosorbent test
RBC	red blood cell
REM	rapid eye movement
RES	reticuloendothelial system
RFFIT	rapid fluorescent focus inhibition test
RFTs	renal function tests
RHD	rheumatic heart disease
RNA	ribonucleic acid
RNP	ribonucleoprotein
RPR	rapid plasma reagin
RR	respiratory rate
RSV	respiratory syncytial virus
RUQ	right upper quadrant
RV	residual volume
Sao_2	oxygen saturation in arterial blood
SBFT	small bowel follow-through
SCC	squamous cell carcinoma
SCID	severe combined immunodeficiency
SERM	selective estrogen receptor modulator
SGOT	serum glutamic-oxaloacetic transaminase
SIADH	syndrome of inappropriate antidiuretic hormone
SIDS	sudden infant death syndrome
SLE	systemic lupus erythematosus
SMA	superior mesenteric artery
SSPE	subacute sclerosing panencephalitis
SSRI	selective serotonin reuptake inhibitor
ST	stable toxin
STD	sexually transmitted disease
T2W	T2-weighted (MRI)
T_3	triiodothyronine
T_4	thyroxine
TAH-BSO	total abdominal hysterectomy–bilateral salpingo-oophorectomy
TB	tuberculosis
TCA	tricyclic antidepressant

TCC	transitional cell carcinoma
TDT	terminal deoxytransferase
TFTs	thyroid function tests
TGF	transforming growth factor
THC	tetrahydrocannabinol
TIA	transient ischemic attack
TLC	total lung capacity
TMP-SMX	trimethoprim-sulfamethoxazole
tPA	tissue plasminogen activator
TP-HA	*Treponema pallidum* hemagglutination assay
TPP	thiamine pyrophosphate
TRAP	tartrate-resistant acid phosphatase
tRNA	transfer ribonucleic acid
TSH	thyroid-stimulating hormone
TSS	toxic shock syndrome
TTP	thrombotic thrombocytopenic purpura
TURP	transurethral resection of the prostate
TXA	thromboxane A
UA	urinalysis
UDCA	ursodeoxycholic acid
UGI	upper GI
UPPP	uvulopalatopharyngoplasty
URI	upper respiratory infection
US	ultrasound
UTI	urinary tract infection
UV	ultraviolet
VDRL	Venereal Disease Research Laboratory
VIN	vulvar intraepithelial neoplasia
VIP	vasoactive intestinal polypeptide
VLDL	very low density lipoprotein
VMA	vanillylmandelic acid
V/Q	ventilation/perfusion (ratio)
VRE	vancomycin-resistant enterococcus
VS	vital signs
VSD	ventricular septal defect
vWF	von Willebrand's factor
VZV	varicella-zoster virus
WAGR	Wilms' tumor, aniridia, genitourinary abnormalities, mental retardation (syndrome)
WBC	white blood cell
WHI	Women's Health Initiative
WPW	Wolff-Parkinson-White syndrome
XR	x-ray
ZN	Ziehl-Neelsen (stain)

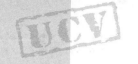

CASE 1

ID/CC A 45-year-old white female is rushed to the OR because of **shock** due to postoperative bleeding; during intubation, she **vomits and aspirates** that day's breakfast.

HPI She had undergone a cholecystectomy 2 days before and had presented with postoperative bleeding requiring surgical exploration.

PE VS: **tachycardia; tachypnea; fever; hypotension**. PE: **central cyanosis**; warm, moist skin; **intercostal retraction; inspiratory crepitant rales** heard over both lung fields.

Labs CBC/PBS: marked **leukocytosis** with neutrophilia; fragmented RBCs; thrombocytopenia. ABGs: **severe hypoxemia with no improvement on 100% oxygen**; ratio of arterial Po_2 to inspired fraction of O_2 < 200. Increased BUN and creatinine; increased AST and ALT.

Imaging CXR: typical **diffuse and symmetric parahilar ("bat-wing" pattern) alveolar filling** process suggestive of **noncardiogenic pulmonary edema**.

Gross Pathology Formation of **hyaline membranes** with proteinaceous deposits in alveoli; **pulmonary edema** with red, heavy lungs which, combined with **widespread atelectasis**, produce **stiff lung** with fibrosis.

Micro Pathology Endothelial and alveolocapillary damage with edema, hyaline membrane formation, and inflammatory infiltrate; **loss of surfactant** with fibroblast activity in later stages.

Treatment Mechanical ventilation with moderate to high levels of positive end-expiratory pressure; antibiotics, steroids, close monitoring of hemodynamic function.

Discussion Adult respiratory distress syndrome is a condition that is associated with **high mortality**; it is caused by gram-negative **sepsis, massive trauma**, burns, disseminated intravascular coagulation (DIC), acute pancreatitis, narcotic overdose, and near-drowning. It is characterized by diffuse alveolar capillary injury, which leads to an increase in vascular permeability and pulmonary edema.

ARDS

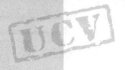

CASE 2

ID/CC

A 65-year-old male presents with **progressively increasing cough and dyspnea** on exertion.

HPI

He is a **retired construction worker** and has a nearly **100-pack-year smoking** history.

PE

VS: normal. PE: grade II **clubbing**; fine crackles auscultated bilaterally over lung bases.

Labs

CBC: normal. PFTs: mixed obstructive and restrictive disease pattern; reduced DL_{CO}. Microscopic exam of sputum reveals **golden-brown beaded rods** (ASBESTOS BODIES) composed of asbestos fibers coated with an iron-containing proteinaceous material.

Imaging

CXR: irregular linear, **interstitial infiltrates** in lower lobes with circumscribed radiopaque densities (PLEURAL PLAQUES). CT (high resolution): posterior and lateral pleura thickened with **calcified plaques** seen bilaterally.

Gross Pathology

Diffuse pulmonary **interstitial fibrosis** with **bilateral pleural calcification** and thickening and involvement of the diaphragm.

Micro Pathology

Calcium-containing dense pleural opacities and plaques of collagen; asbestos bodies.

Treatment

Supportive and symptomatic treatment (oxygen, bronchodilators, antibiotics); **prevention of further exposure**; **smoking cessation**; counseling regarding **high risk** of **bronchogenic carcinoma** and **malignant mesothelioma**.

Discussion

Prolonged exposure to asbestos in significantly cumulative doses results in **pulmonary parenchymal scarring**. This process is self-perpetuating, but cessation of exposure may slow disease progression. Complications include **bronchogenic carcinoma, malignant mesothelioma, cor pulmonale, and death**; smoking and asbestos exposure **synergistically** increase cancer risk.

asbestos

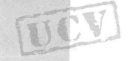

CASE 3

ID/CC	A 10-year-old girl is brought into the ER in **acute respiratory distress**.
HPI	The patient is known to be **allergic to cats and pollen**; her mother states that she had a **recent URI**. She also complains of a history of moderate **intermittent dyspnea that is exacerbated by exercise**.
PE	VS: no fever; **tachypnea** (RR 32); BP: normal. PE: inspiratory and **expiratory wheezes** (due to bronchoconstriction, small airway inflammation); boggy and pale nasal mucosa; **accessory muscle** use during breathing; enlarged chest AP diameter; **hyperresonant** to percussion.
Labs	ABGs: primary respiratory alkalosis (hyperventilation). CBC: **eosinophilia** (13%). PFTs: low FEV_1/FVC.
Imaging	CXR: hyperinflation with flattened diaphragms (increased residual volume due to **air trapping**); peribronchial cuffing.
Gross Pathology	**Hyperinflation** with air trapping in alveoli; **plugs of inspissated mucus**; edema of mucosal lining.
Micro Pathology	Inflammatory infiltrate of bronchial epithelium, mainly eosinophilic; plugging of airways **with thickened mucus** (CURSCHMANN'S SPIRALS); hypertrophy of mucous glands; elongated rhomboid crystals derived from eosinophil cytoplasm (CHARCOT–LEYDEN CRYSTALS); hyperplasia of smooth muscle of bronchi.
Treatment	Nebulized bronchodilators, parenteral steroids, and ventilatory support for acute exacerbations; inhaled bronchodilators and steroids for chronic, persistent symptoms; mast cell stabilizers such as cromolyn and leukotriene inhibitors such as zafirlukast for prophylaxis.
Discussion	Bronchial asthma is characterized by **hyperreactivity of the airways and obstruction due to bronchospasm, edema, and mucus**. It is also known as **reactive airway disease**.

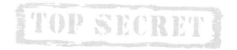

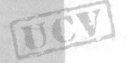

CASE 4

ID/CC	A 50-year-old white male develops a **fever 24 hours after surgery**.
HPI	He underwent an emergency **laparotomy** for a perforated peptic ulcer without any intraoperative or immediate postoperative complications.
PE	VS: **fever**; BP normal; **tachypnea**; **tachycardia**. PE: no cyanosis; **scattered rales** and **decreased breath sounds**; no calf tenderness; no hematoma or discharge from wound; no inflammation of IV line veins; no urinary symptoms.
Labs	ABGs: mild **hypoxemia**. CBC: slight neutrophilic leukocytosis. Blood and sputum culture sterile. ECG: sinus tachycardia.
Imaging	CXR: **dense opacity in right lower lobe** (collapsed lobe) with elevation of right hemidiaphragm (due to volume loss).
Treatment	Chest physiotherapy (incentive spirometry); deep inspirations; mucolytic agents.
Discussion	Postoperative atelectasis is the most common cause of postoperative fever in the first 48 hours; alveolar collapse is produced by occlusion due to viscid secretions favored by recumbency, hypoventilation, and over-sedation. Other causes of postoperative fever, usually seen later in the postoperative period, include UTI, IV catheter infection, deep venous thrombosis, wound infection, and drug reactions.

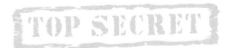

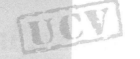

CASE 5

ID/CC
A 14-year-old male presents with complaints of **exertional dyspnea, chronic productive cough**, and **occasional hemoptysis**.

HPI
He was diagnosed with **cystic fibrosis** at age 4 and has had **recurrent pulmonary infections** requiring frequent hospitalizations.

PE
VS: low-grade fever (38°C); tachycardia (HR 110); tachypnea (RR 28). PE: pallor and grade II **clubbing** noted; **coarse crackles** auscultated over both lung fields.

Labs
CBC: **normocytic, normochromic anemia**; low hematocrit. Sputum culture reveals *Staphylococcus aureus*. PFTs: decreased FEV_1/FVC suggestive of obstructive pathology.

Imaging
XR, chest: increased bronchovascular markings; honeycomb appearance (due to end-on shadows of dilated bronchioles); loss of lung volume (atelectasis). CT (high resolution), chest: **dilated bronchioles with "signet ring" appearance** (due to adjacent branch of pulmonary artery).

Gross Pathology
Long, tubelike, irreversibly dilated bronchioles extending to the pleura with loss of lung parenchyma.

Treatment
Supportive measures; antibiotics; bronchodilators, expectorants, and **physical therapy** to promote bronchial drainage. Surgery may be indicated for localized or segmental bronchiectasis or when medical therapy fails.

Discussion
Dilatation of the bronchial tree leads to infections and to further irreversible dilatation. Underlying causes include **obstruction** due to tumor, foreign bodies, and mucus impaction; **congenital disorders** such as Kartagener's syndrome, Williams-Campbell syndrome, and **cystic fibrosis**; and **infections** due to *Bordetella pertussis*, togavirus, RSV, measles, and *Mycobacterium tuberculosis*. **Complications** include **lung abscesses, metastatic brain abscesses, amyloidosis, and cor pulmonale.**

bronchiectasis

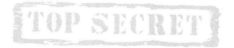

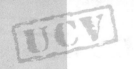

ID/CC   A **60-year-old male** is referred to an allergist for late-onset **asthma** that has been **unresponsive to bronchodilators and antibiotics.**

HPI   He has also been having chest pain (ANGINA), fatigue, anorexia, and pain in both calves (CLAUDICATION) on exertion that are of recent onset.

PE   VS: tachypnea; mild fever; **mild hypertension** (BP 150/100) (secondary to renal vascular involvement). PE: marked respiratory distress; widespread **wheezes** bilaterally; numerous **purpuric lesions on feet** (due to cutaneous small vessel vasculitis).

Labs   CBC: mild anemia; leukocytosis (> 10,000/μL); Hct < 35%; thrombocytosis (> 400,000/μL); **eosinophilia (> 1000/μL). Elevated BUN and creatinine;** P-ANCA positive; elevated ESR and C-reactive protein. UA: **proteinuria;** presence of **RBCs, WBCs, and granular casts.** PFTs: FEV_1/FVC ratio reduced (**obstructive pulmonary disease**). ECG: sinus tachycardia.

Imaging   CXR: **bilateral upper and lower lobe infiltrates** and noncavitating nodules.

Gross Pathology   Lung shows hemorrhagic infarcts secondary to thrombi in affected arteries.

Micro Pathology   Transbronchial lung biopsy shows **granulomatous lesions in vascular and extravascular sites accompanied by intense eosinophilia;** skin biopsy of purpuric lesions shows **vasculitic lesions**—fibrinoid necrosis of media with mixture of inflammatory cells extending along adventitia; occasional aneurysms and secondary thromboses seen; the arterial internal elastic lamina is destroyed and intima and media are thickened.

Treatment   **Prednisone** is effective in inducing remission; **cyclophosphamide** or other cytotoxic/immunosuppressive agents when disease is **refractory** to steroids; monitor disease course using **ESR levels.**

Discussion   Churg–Strauss syndrome is an idiopathic systemic **small- and medium-vessel granulomatous vasculitis** (grouped with polyarteritis nodosa [PAN], which does not involve lungs) that is characterized by a triad of late-onset **asthma,** a fluctuating **eosinophilia,** and an **extrapulmonary vasculitis.**

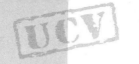

ID/CC A 50-year-old white male **smoker** presents with **productive cough, copious sputum**, shortness of breath, and **fever**.

HPI The patient has a **40-pack-year** smoking history. He has also experienced chronic dyspnea on exertion; chronic **productive cough**, usually **in the mornings**, for several years; and multiple colds each winter.

PE VS: fever. PE: stocky build with plethora; wheezes.

Labs CBC: elevated WBC count (14,000); neutrophils predominant; **secondary polycythemia**. *Streptococcus pneumoniae* or *Haemophilus influenzae* on Gram stain of sputum sample. ABGs: decreased Po_2; elevated Pco_2. PFTs: decreased vital capacity; **decreased FEV_1**.

Imaging CXR: increased bronchovascular markings in lower lung fields.

Gross Pathology Thick mucous secretion; edema of bronchial mucosa.

Micro Pathology **Increased size and number of mucous glands** (Reid's index > 50); inflammation; fibrosis; squamous metaplasia.

Treatment Antibiotics; bronchodilators; steroids; oxygen; smoking cessation.

COPD – chronic bronchitis

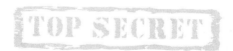

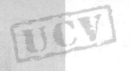

ID/CC   A 55-year-old male complains of progressively increasing **shortness of breath on exertion** for the past few months.

HPI   He also complains of a nonproductive mild cough and has a **40-pack-year smoking history** but has no history of hemoptysis or occupational exposure to inorganic or organic dusts.

PE   VS: moderate tachypnea. PE: moderate respiratory distress; **using accessory muscles of respiration**; fullness of neck veins during expiration; chest **barrel-shaped**; percussion note hyperresonant; **cardiac and liver dullness** are **obliterated**; scattered rhonchi bilaterally; **heart sounds heard distant** but normal.

Labs   ABGs: mild hypoxia with respiratory alkalosis. PFTs: increased residual volume; **decreased FEV_1/FVC ratio** (OBSTRUCTIVE DISEASE PATTERN); decreased DL_{CO}.

Imaging   CXR (PA view): **hyperlucent lung fields with a few bullae**; flattening of diaphragm and elongated tubular heart shadow.

Gross Pathology   Air spaces dilated; **upper lobes most affected.**

Micro Pathology   Pattern of **centrilobular emphysema**: alveolar septa are visibly diminished in number along with increased air spaces.

Treatment   Cessation of smoking, bronchodilators, steroids in resistant cases, antibiotics during acute exacerbations, and home oxygen therapy.

Discussion   Emphysema is defined as abnormal permanent enlargement of the air spaces distal to the terminal bronchiole accompanied by the destruction of the alveolar walls; emphysema may involve the acinus and the lobule uniformly in a pattern called panacinar, or it may primarily involve the respiratory bronchioles, termed centriacinar. Panacinar emphysema is common in patients with α_1-antitrypsin deficiency. Centriacinar emphysema is commonly found in cigarette smokers and is rare in non-smokers; it is usually more extensive and severe in the upper lobes.

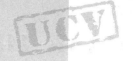

CASE 9

ID/CC

A 58-year-old male complains of **headache**, anxiety, shortness of breath, and increased sleepiness (SOMNOLENCE) while experiencing an **acute exacerbation of COPD**.

HPI

The patient is a **chronic smoker** and also complains of recent **blurring of vision**. He has a history of episodic shortness of breath, mucoid cough, and occasional wheezing (consistent with predominantly **bronchitic COPD**) but no history of neurologic deficit, previous hypertension, or diabetes.

PE

VS: tachycardia; tachypnea; mild systolic hypertension; no fever. PE: anxious and in moderate respiratory distress; using accessory muscles of respiration with prolonged expiration; mild **central cyanosis and pallor; no clubbing**; extremities warm; **flapping tremor of hand** (ASTERIXIS); **bounding pulses** (due to high volume); funduscopy reveals **early papilledema**; chest barrel-shaped with bilateral rhonchi and occasional rales; no focal neurologic deficits.

Labs

ABGs: **hypoxia, hypercapnia, and partially compensated respiratory acidosis**. CBC: polycythemia.

Imaging

CXR (PA view): increased bronchovascular markings (dirty lung fields).

Treatment

Low-dose continuous oxygen inhalation and, if required, **mechanical ventilation** to reverse acidosis; broad-spectrum antibiotics, bronchodilators (ipratropium bromide and sympathomimetics), and steroids are used in COPD patients.

Discussion

Dyspnea and headache are the cardinal symptoms of hypercapnia. Hypercapnia also produces a variety of neurologic abnormalities; symptoms include somnolence, blurred vision, restlessness, and anxiety that can progress to tremors, asterixis, delirium, and coma. Supplemental oxygen should be used sparingly to avoid increasing PaO_2, which removes the hypoxic respiratory stimulus and leads to respiratory depression.

Carbon dioxide narcosis

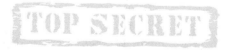

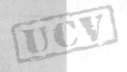
ID/CC   A 37-year-old **male** in the ICU develops **petechiae, altered sensorium, and marked dyspnea** that prove refractory to oxygen therapy.

HPI   Twenty-four hours ago, he was admitted to the hospital with **fractures of the shafts of both femurs, the pelvis, and the right humerus,** sustained following a fall from a 20-foot-high stepladder.

PE   VS: fever; marked dyspnea. PE: **delirium; central cyanosis;** using accessory muscles of respiration; wheezing heard over both lung fields.

Labs   ABGs: **profound arterial hypoxemia with hypercapnia.** CBC/PBS: thrombocytopenia. **Fat demonstrated in urine and sputum;** normal PT and PTT.

Imaging   CXR: early, normal; later, bilateral perihilar ("BAT-WING") appearance of **pulmonary infiltrates** without cardiomegaly (due to noncardiogenic pulmonary edema). XR, plain: long bone fractures.

Micro Pathology   Obstruction of pulmonary vessels by fat globules; chemical pneumonitis.

Treatment   Intermittent positive pressure ventilation with 100% oxygen, supportive management.

Discussion   Fat embolization usually occurs **24 to 72 hours after fractures of the shafts of the long bones**.

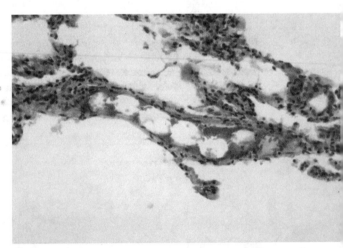

Figure 010 Fat globules evident as empty circular spaces within a small pulmonary vessel.

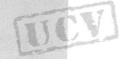

CASE 11

ID/CC A 50-year-old **farmer** presents with severe **shortness of breath** (DYSPNEA) and **fatigue**.

HPI He also complains of a **dry cough** and **mild fever**. His symptoms are exacerbated when he works in the fields, especially when he comes into contact with **moldy hay**. He does not smoke and drinks alcohol occasionally.

PE VS: tachycardia; tachypnea; mild fever. PE: moderate respiratory distress; scattered rhonchi and **bilateral fine rales**.

Labs CBC: leukocytosis with shift to left. Elevated ESR; **serum antibodies against thermophilic *Actinomyces* organisms**; bronchoalveolar lavage shows marked lymphocytosis, primarily suppressor-cytotoxic T cells. PFTs: **restrictive lung disease** pattern.

Imaging CXR: bilateral **reticulonodular infiltrates with fibrosis**. CT: areas of ground-glass abnormalities with centrilobular peribronchial nodules.

Gross Pathology Fibrosis with honeycombing.

Micro Pathology Bronchoscopic lung biopsy reveals interstitial pneumonia with lymphocytes and plasma cells in alveolar walls as well as scattered focal granulomas with foreign body giant cells.

Treatment Environmental control to minimize antigen exposure; steroids.

Discussion Hypersensitivity pneumonitis (allergic alveolitis) refers to interstitial lung disease that results from inhalation of organic antigens. Hypersensitivity pneumonitis is believed to have an immunologic basis (e.g., cytotoxic, immune complex, and cell-mediated reactions); **the most common form of hypersensitivity pneumonitis, called farmer's lung, is caused by inhalation of a thermophilic *Actinomyces* organism present in moldy hay and grain.** Other common causes of hypersensitivity pneumonitis include pigeon breeder's disease and bird fancier's disease, in which inhaled serum proteins from pigeons or parakeets induce the syndrome. Humidifier lung disease results from exposure to contaminated forced-air systems.

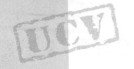

CASE 12

ID/CC A 65-year-old male complains of progressive shortness of breath on exertion and a chronic **dry cough**.

HPI The patient has **never smoked** cigarettes and has no history of exposure to occupational dusts or fumes; he has not had a productive cough or hemoptysis.

PE VS: warm but **cyanosed**; tachycardia (HR 108); tachypnea; BP normal. PE: **clubbing present**; JVP not elevated; heart sounds normal with no additional sounds or murmurs; respiratory examination reveals presence of bilateral **basal fine inspiratory crepitations**.

Labs ABGs: hypoxemia. PFTs: **decreased DL$_{CO}$**; desaturation with exercise; proportionately reduced FEV$_1$ and FVC so that ratio remained unchanged (due to restrictive disease). Bronchoalveolar lavage predominantly neutrophilic; serum calcium and ACE levels low.

Imaging CXR: reticulonodular shadows in both lower lung fields with occasional areas of "**honeycombing**." CT (high resolution): fibrosis in lower lung lobes suggestive of usual **interstitial pneumonitis pattern of IPF**.

Micro Pathology Bronchoscopically obtained lung biopsy reveals presence of fibrosis, inflammatory round cell infiltrate, and thickening of the alveolar septa.

Treatment Systemic steroids.

Discussion The main differential diagnoses to consider are lung fibrosis associated with a connective tissue disorder (rule out by history and clinical exam), extrinsic alveolitis due to organic dusts, left-sided heart failure, sarcoidosis (rule out on the basis of absence of any other system involvement, normal calcium and ACE levels, negative Kveim's test, and lack of hilar lymphadenopathy observed on CXR), lymphangitis carcinomatosa (rule out on biopsy and CT), and pneumoconiosis. The onset of idiopathic pulmonary fibrosis is typically in the fifth or sixth decade.

IPF

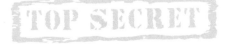

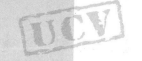

ID/CC	A 58-year-old male presents with **shortness of breath** (DYSPNEA), **hoarseness, cough,** and **hemoptysis.**
HPI	He has an **80-pack-year smoking history.** Over the past 2 months, he has also had a **significant loss of appetite and weight.**
PE	Marked pallor; **cachexia; clubbing;** mild wheezing at rest; chest barrel shaped (emphysematous) and movements diminished on right; **dullness to percussion** over right middle lobe; **no breath sounds** heard over right middle lobe; vocal fremitus reduced in same area.
Labs	CBC: **normocytic, normochromic anemia.** Gram and ZN stains of sputum for acid-fast bacilli negative; sputum cytology reveals presence of **malignant squamous cells.**
Imaging	CXR/CT: irregular hilar mass on right side, producing an obstruction atelectasis of right middle lobe. Bronchoscopy: right-sided hilar mass obstructing right middle bronchus.
Gross Pathology	Postsurgical specimen reveals an irregular invasive mass of grayish-tan tumor spreading out from right middle bronchus and obstructing it.
Micro Pathology	Biopsy reveals presence of malignant squamous cells, cellular stratification, **intercellular bridges,** and "keratin pearls."
Treatment	Surgical resection can be potentially curative in patients with no involvement of surrounding mediastinal structures, contralateral lymph nodes, or distant organs; chemotherapy and/or radiation therapy may be useful in management of unresectable disease.
Discussion	Lung cancer is the **most preventable cancer.** Owing to the increased incidence of smoking, lung cancer has exceeded breast cancer as the leading cause of cancer death in women. A **Pancoast's tumor** is a lung tumor located at the lung apex in the superior pulmonary sulcus that causes compression of the cervical sympathetic plexus, resulting in **Horner's syndrome** (ptosis, miosis, anhidrosis) as well as scapular pain and ulnar nerve radiculopathy.

lung carcinoma (squamous cell)

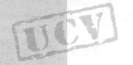

CASE 14

ID/CC	A 67-year-old male is referred to a clinic for evaluation of **pleuritic pain**, **weight loss**, gradually progressive **dyspnea**, and a **nonproductive cough** of a few months' duration.
HPI	He worked in a **shipyard** for 20 years before retiring, an occupation that involved **asbestos exposure**.
PE	VS: normal. PS: **clubbing of fingers**; mild cyanosis; **reduced chest expansion**; end-inspiratory rales auscultated over both lung fields; **dull percussion, reduced breath sounds**, and egophony in right side (due to pleural effusion).
Labs	CBC/PBS: polycythemia; **marked eosinophilia**. PFTs: **restrictive pattern** observed (decreased vital capacity and decreased total lung capacity with normal FEV_1/FVC ratio). Reduced diffusion capacity; pleural effusion bloody and shows acidic pH (< 7.3).
Imaging	CXR: right-sided pleural effusion; diffuse bilateral **interstitial fibrosis**; **parietal pleural calcifications**. CT: highly irregular pleural-based masses; hemorrhagic effusion.
Gross Pathology	Thick, **fibrous pleural plaques with calcification**; diffuse interstitial fibrosis; asbestos compounds form nest for further deposition of iron salts and glycoproteins (FERRUGINOUS ASBESTOS BODIES).
Micro Pathology	Epithelioid pattern of pleural malignant sarcomatous transformation with cellular atypia and high mitotic index.
Treatment	Surgery, chemotherapy, radiation therapy, and multimodality treatments may be employed; poor prognosis.
Discussion	Occupational exposure to asbestos is found in 80% of cases of malignant mesothelioma; it produces lung fibrosis with a restrictive pattern. Asbestos and tobacco exposure synergistically increase the risk of lung adenocarcinoma.

malignant mesothelioma

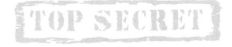

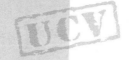

ID/CC

A 37-year-old female comes to the emergency room complaining of **pleuritic pain** on the right side of her chest and **dyspnea** together with fever and a productive cough.

HPI

There is no hemoptysis. The pain is typically **sharp and stabbing**, and it arises when she takes a deep breath (PLEURISY).

PE

Decreased chest movement during inhalation on right side; **dullness** on percussion of right lung base; **reduced or absent breath sounds** over right lung base; bronchial breath sounds auscultated on right side; friction rub; location of **dullness moves with respiration; decreased tactile fremitus** over right lung.

Labs

CBC: elevated WBC count with predominance of neutrophils. Gram-positive diplococci on sputum smear and culture; **elevated protein, decreased glucose, and many neutrophils in pleural exudate.**

Imaging

CXR: pleural effusion on right side. XR, lateral decubitus: **layering of fluid** (therefore not loculated).

Treatment

Antibiotics and needle drainage of effusion (THORACENTESIS); sometimes obliteration of pleural space.

Discussion

Pleural effusions may be due to infection (viral, bacterial, mycobacterial, fungal); other causes are malignancies, congestive heart failure, cirrhosis, nephrotic syndrome, trauma, pancreatitis, collagen diseases, and drug reactions. Effusions may be **transudative** (< 3 g/dL of protein) or **exudative** (> 3 g/dL of protein). Elevated pleural fluid LDH levels may be suggestive of malignancy. **Transudative** pleural effusions are commonly caused by congestive heart failure, cirrhosis, and nephrotic syndrome, whereas **exudative** pleural effusions are caused by TB, infections, malignancy, pancreatitis, pulmonary embolus, and chylothorax (milky pleural fluid).

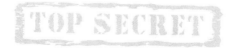

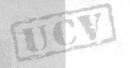

ID/CC   A 25-year-old white **male** complains of **sudden pleuritic chest pain** and **shortness of breath** that **awakens him at night**.

HPI   He **smokes** one pack of cigarettes a day and states that his paternal **uncle once had a similar episode**.

PE   **Tall, thin** patient; diaphoretic and feels weak; left chest expands poorly on inspiration; trachea and apex beat displaced to right; left side **hyperresonant** to percussion; **decreased breath sounds; decreased tactile fremitus**.

Labs   ABGs: decreased Po_2; elevated Pco_2.

Imaging   CXR: partial collapse of left lung with no lung markings except **thin line parallel to chest wall**; costophrenic sulcus abnormally radiolucent ("DEEP SULCUS" SIGN) in supine film.

Gross Pathology   Types: traumatic, spontaneous, tension, open; common causes: surgical puncture, rupture of emphysematous bullae, positive pressure mechanical ventilation, bronchopleural fistula.

Treatment   Pneumothorax evacuation via pleural catheter (CHEST TUBE).

Discussion   The usual cause of spontaneous pneumothorax is rupture of a subpleural bleb.

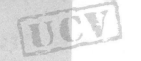

CASE 17

ID/CC
A 40-year-old male is brought to the ER with complaints of **sudden-onset, severe right-sided chest pain followed by severe difficulty breathing.**

HPI
He is a chronic smoker and has predominantly **emphysematous** COPD.

PE
VS: severe tachycardia; tachypnea; hypotension; no fever. PE: **cyanosis; trachea shifted** to left; chest exam reveals **hyperresonant percussion note on right, diminished breath sounds,** and **decreased tactile fremitus.**

Labs
ABGs: hypoxemia; respiratory alkalosis. ECG: normal.

Imaging
CXR (after patient stabilizes): **right pneumothorax compressing lung parenchyma and shifting of mediastinum toward left.** Flattened left hemidiaphragm.

Gross Pathology
Pleural space is filled with air and lung is atelectatic (to demonstrate pneumothorax at autopsy, the chest cavity is opened under water, letting air bubbles escape).

Micro Pathology
Section of lung shows collapsed alveolar spaces.

Treatment
Immediate life-saving treatment consists of inserting a wide-bore IV cannula in the second intercostal space on the affected side to decompress the pleural cavity if a chest drain is not immediately available; the wide-bore needle can then be replaced by a chest drain connected to an underwater seal.

Discussion
In tension pneumothorax, air enters the pleural space during inspiration and is prevented from escaping during expiration (because an airway or tissue flap acts as a one-way valve); there is a progressive increase in pleural air, which is under pressure (i.e., tension). Tension pneumothorax occurs in only 1% to 2% of cases of idiopathic spontaneous pneumothorax; it is a more common manifestation of the barotrauma that may occur during positive pressure mechanical ventilation. Risk factors for spontaneous pneumothorax include COPD, cystic fibrosis, asthma, and tuberculosis.

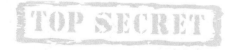

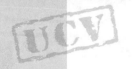

CASE 18

ID/CC	A **34-year-old** white obese **female** complains of **shortness of breath**, dizziness, and near-fainting spells.
HPI	She has been taking **prescription medication** for approximately 6 months in order to **lose weight**.
PE	Obesity; mild cyanosis; **large "a" wave** in jugular venous pressure; parasternal heave; **loud S2**; narrow splitting of S2; rales on both bases; hepatomegaly.
Labs	CBC: **polycythemia**. ECG: **right-axis deviation; right ventricle and right atrial hypertrophy**. ABGs: hypoxemia.
Imaging	CXR: enlarged right ventricle; enlarged main pulmonary artery with peripheral pruning.
Gross Pathology	Enlarged right ventricle with myocardial fiber hypertrophy; atherosclerosis of pulmonary artery; narrowing of arterioles.
Micro Pathology	Atheromas in main elastic arteries. Thickening of the media and intima in medium size muscular arteries, causing near-obliteration of the lumen.
Treatment	Calcium channel blockers; prostacyclin; endothelin receptor antagonists; inhaled nitric oxide; heart-lung transplantation can be considered.
Discussion	Primary pulmonary hypertension is a pathologic increase in pulmonary artery pressure; if long-standing, it causes fatal right heart failure. It may be primary (idiopathic) or secondary to intrinsic pulmonary disease.

Figure 018 Hypertrophic and dilated right ventricle.

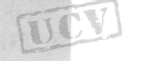

CASE 19

ID/CC A 60-year-old female who had undergone right **total hip replacement** presents on the sixth postoperative day with central **chest pain** and **acute-onset dyspnea.**

HPI She has been **immobile** since the surgery.

PE VS: low-grade fever; tachycardia; **tachypnea**; hypotension. PE: central cyanosis; **elevated JVP**; **right ventricular gallop rhythm with widely split S2.**

Labs ABGs: **hypoxia and hypercapnia** (type 2 respiratory failure). ECG: **S1Q3T3** pattern and sinus **tachycardia.** Positive D-dimer test.

Imaging CXR: right lower lobe atelectasis. V/Q: three areas of ventilation-perfusion mismatch in right lung. Spiral CT, chest: filling defect in right main pulmonary artery suggestive of an occlusive embolus. Angio, pulmonary: confirmatory; not required if V/Q scan is high probability. US, Doppler: **clot in right common femoral vein.**

Gross Pathology Large thrombus seen in pulmonary artery.

Micro Pathology Large occlusive thrombus seen in pulmonary artery with variable degree of recanalization.

Treatment Supportive; thrombolytic therapy; consider embolectomy; heparin, Coumadin, and low-molecular-weight heparin (enoxaparin) instituted for prophylaxis (monitor INR).

Discussion Pulmonary emboli most commonly originate from proximal deep venous thrombosis. Pulmonary angiography is the gold standard in the diagnosis of pulmonary embolism, but obtain a V/Q scan initially if clinically suspected. **Virchow's triad** outlines the risk factors for thrombus formation and includes **blood stasis** (e.g., immobilization), **endothelial damage** (e.g., surgery), and **hypercoagulable states** (e.g., malignancy, pregnancy, severe burns). **Large emboli** may cause cardiovascular collapse and sudden death.

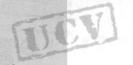

CASE 20

ID/CC	A 28-year-old black female complains of fever, dyspnea, arthralgia, and erythematous, tender nodules on both legs.
HPI	She has no history of foreign travel or contact with a tubercular patient.
PE	VS: fever. PE: tender, erythematous nodules over extensor aspects of both legs (ERYTHEMA NODOSUM); arthralgias of both knees; splenomegaly.
Labs	CBC: lymphopenia; eosinophilia. Lytes: elevated serum calcium; hypercalciuria. ACE levels elevated; blood cultures negative; Mantoux test negative; fungal serology negative. PFTs: evidence of restrictive changes. Transbronchial lung biopsy ordered.
Imaging	CXR: bilateral hilar lymphadenopathy and right paratracheal adenopathy; interstitial infiltrates; no pleural effusion.
Gross Pathology	Firm nodules only a few millimeters in size in affected organs; can become confluent and give rise to larger nodules.
Micro Pathology	Lymph node biopsy reveals noncaseating granulomas with fibrotic acellular core surrounded by lymphocytes, epithelioid cells, and Langerhan's giant cells.
Treatment	Corticosteroids.
Discussion	In the United States, the incidence of sarcoidosis is highest in black women, with onset between 20 and 40 years of age. The disease may be asymptomatic; however, symptoms may be constitutional and may involve many different organ systems, including the lungs, lymph nodes, skin, eye, upper respiratory tract, reticuloendothelial system, liver, kidneys, nervous system, and heart. Approximately 60% to 70% of sarcoidosis patients recover with few or no residual symptoms.

TOP SECRET

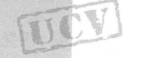

ID/CC A 56-year-old male presents with progressively increasing **dyspnea** and **dry cough** of several years' duration.

HPI He is a nonsmoker, but his occupational history includes **mining and quarrying**.

PE No clubbing, cyanosis, or lymphadenopathy; **reduced chest expansion** on inspiration; **dry inspiratory crackles** auscultated in upper lobes of both lungs.

Labs PFTs: combined **obstructive and restrictive pattern** of functional impairment. Bronchoscopically-guided lung biopsy establishes diagnosis; negative Mantoux test; sputum cytology and staining for acid-fast bacilli negative.

Imaging CXR, PA: rounded small opacities in upper lobes with retraction and **hilar lymphadenopathy**; **"eggshell" calcification of lymph nodes**.

Gross Pathology Dense, small collagenous nodules in the upper lungs in the early stages; spread and become more diffuse as disease progresses.

Micro Pathology Hyalinized whorls of collagen with little or no inflammation; polarized light demonstrates silica particles within nodules.

Treatment Supportive; avoidance of further exposure.

Discussion There is an **increased incidence of tuberculosis** in silicosis patients. Silicosis leads to restrictive lung disease that varies in severity from mild to disabling.

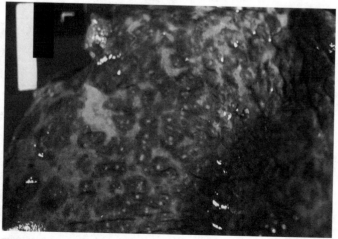

Figure 021 Dense, small, blackened nodules just under the pleural surface of the lung.

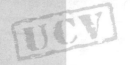

CASE 22

ID/CC   A 45-year-old Hispanic female is brought to the gynecologist for an evaluation of a **gross difference in the size of her breasts** of recent origin.

HPI   Her medical history is unremarkable. Despite the recent increase in the size of her right breast, she **does not feel any pain and feels only a sensation of fullness**.

PE   **Very large mass** with firm, "wooden-log" consistency involving almost all of right breast, making it twice the size of opposite breast; **mobile mass**; appears **well circumscribed**; collateral bluish veins seen on skin along with striae; no peau d'orange appearance; no nipple retraction, axillary lymphadenopathy, or hepatomegaly; opposite breast normal.

Imaging   US: large, smooth multilobulated mass.

Gross Pathology   Large tumor with numerous **cystic spaces on cut section of stroma, producing recesses and longitudinal openings** and causing a leaflike (**phyllodes**) appearance.

Micro Pathology   Abundance of normal-looking ducts, acini, and stroma with no signs of cellular atypia and low mitotic index.

Treatment   Wide local excision with a rim of normal breast tissue or mastectomy.

Discussion   A less common benign tumor of breast that is also known as giant fibroadenoma, cystosarcoma phyllodes is a **bulky tumor** that, although usually benign histologically, **may recur** following excision and sometimes undergoes malignant degeneration (5% to 10%). It **rarely metastasizes** to lymph nodes or distant sites.

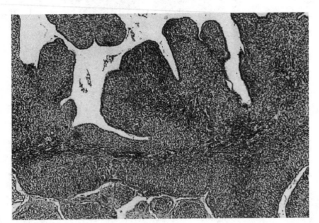

Figure 022 Cellular stroma with high mitotic rate and epithelial lined leaf-like architecture.

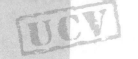

CASE 23

ID/CC

A 27-year-old **woman** who is **actively training** for a marathon notes a **painful lump** in the upper outer quadrant of her right breast of 2 days' duration.

HPI

She has no history of fever and no known family history of breast cancer.

PE

Retraction of overlying skin in upper outer quadrant of right breast; **indurated lesion** the size of a lemon in same area; axillary lymph nodes not palpable.

Imaging

Mammo: **irregular mass** with **focal areas** of **eggshell calcification**. US: solid, ill-defined mass with altered surrounding architecture.

Gross Pathology

Yellowish, fatty fluid on aspiration.

Micro Pathology

Excisional biopsy shows localized area of **granulation tissue** within which are numerous lipid-laden macrophages subjacent to necrotic fat cells.

Treatment

No other active management required.

Discussion

Fat necrosis of the breast is a unilateral localized process associated with **trauma**, breast biopsy, reduction mammoplasty, and radiation. It is easily confused with cancer due to induration, fibrosis, dystrophic calcification, and retraction of overlying skin; the key distinction is the **presence of pain**. However, biopsy is necessary for definitive diagnosis.

GYN

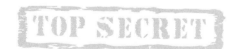

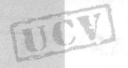

ID/CC   A 32-year-old woman presents with **painful bilateral breast masses**.

HPI   The **pain is cyclic** in nature and **increases in her premenstrual phase**, at which time the **masses enlarge rapidly and then shrink**. She feels that both breasts are nodular and is concerned that she may have cancer.

PE   Mildly tender mass palpable in upper and outer quadrant of right and left breast; both **breasts nodular with multiple thickened areas**; no changes in overlying skin or nipple noted (vs. breast cancer); no axillary lymphadenopathy found.

Labs   Aspiration from breast mass reveals nonbloody fluid; **mass disappears completely after aspiration**.

Imaging   Mammo: nodularity and benign calcifications, no malignant features.

Gross Pathology   Cysts of various sizes ranging from microscopic to several millimeters surrounded by dense fibrotic tissue; contains clear or brown fluid.

Micro Pathology   Proliferation of acini in lobules (SCLEROSING ADENOSIS).

Treatment   Reassurance and symptomatic management.

Discussion   Fibrocystic disease of the breast is common in women between the ages of 35 and 55 and carries an increased risk of invasive breast cancer in patients with epithelial hyperplasia and atypia. Fibrocystic changes may result from hormone imbalances with either an excess of estrogen or a deficiency of progesterone.

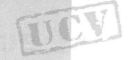
ID/CC

A 59-year-old white female comes to her family doctor because of a presumed "infection" in her right **breast**; she complains of **pain and swelling**.

HPI

Her history is unremarkable.

PE

VS: **no fever** or other systemic sign of infection. PE: right breast warm, **rock-hard, and swollen with no areas** of fluctuation; one-third of breast **erythematous** with shiny overlying skin having **peau d'orange** appearance; **painful** to touch and pressure; several axillary **lymph nodes enlarged** and **firm**; some **coalescent**.

Labs

Routine lab work normal.

Micro Pathology

Large spheroidal cells and fine stroma infiltrated by lymphocytes on breast skin biopsy; lymphatic vessels occluded by tumor cells; immuno-staining positive for overexpression of HER2/neu (associated with poor prognosis).

Treatment

Combined-modality treatment with initial induction chemotherapy followed by surgery and/or radiation.

Discussion

Inflammatory carcinoma of the breast is defined as breast cancer with angiolymphatic spread; it is characterized by a malignant course with early and widespread metastases. Perform skin biopsy in patients diagnosed with breast infection who do not respond promptly to antibiotic treatment.

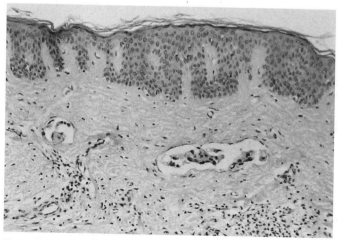

Figure 025 Nodules of breast epithelium surrounded by necrotic adipose tissue with an infiltration of macrophages.

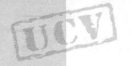

ID/CC A **35-year-old** female rushes to the emergency room and waits to see a doctor because she is concerned about a **bloody nipple discharge** that she discovered this morning.

HPI She exercises, is very health conscious, and always has safe sex.

PE Palpation around left nipple reveals **blood coming from one of the duct openings** and a **small, soft lump** beneath areola; no breast masses or axillary lymphadenopathy.

Imaging Mammo: negative. Ductography: dilated duct with intraluminal filling defect.

Gross Pathology Epithelial papillary growth with fibrotic components, characteristically located **within a lactiferous duct**.

Micro Pathology No cellular atypia or anaplastic changes on specimen of bloody discharge; only blood intermixed with foamy macrophages and benign ductal epithelium with fibrovascular core.

Treatment Surgical resection of lactiferous duct (MICRODOCHECTOMY) followed by histologic examination to rule out carcinoma.

Discussion Papilloma of the breast is a benign proliferation of ductal epithelial tissue and is the most common cause of serous/sanguineous discharge.

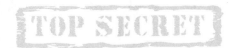

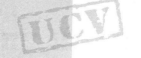

CASE 27

ID/CC	A 46-year-old **woman** presents with a palpable mass in the left breast.
HPI	The patient has been admitted to the hospital to obtain an excisional biopsy and for planning further management. The **patient's older sister recently died of metastatic breast cancer.**
PE	Left breast mass on palpation; nipples normally located without evidence of retraction; no evidence of axillary lymphadenopathy or hepatomegaly.
Imaging	Mammo: frequently normal or an asymmetric density without definable margins.
Gross Pathology	Firm, white, irregularly shaped 3-cm mass was removed from each breast.
Micro Pathology	Histologic sections reveal terminal lobules distended by intermediate-sized cells with scant mitotic activity; neoplastic cells infiltrate the stroma with individual neoplastic cells in a single file (INDIAN FILE PATTERN) that surrounds the terminal lobule in a target-appearing fashion.
Treatment	Modified radical mastectomy with sentinel lymph node biopsy; radiotherapy and adjuvant chemotherapy. Frequent mammographic surveillance is needed owing to the **high incidence of a second primary in the same or opposite breast.**
Discussion	Infiltrating lobular carcinoma is the most common malignancy of the terminal lobule. It accounts for 10% to 13% of all breast cancers.

GYN

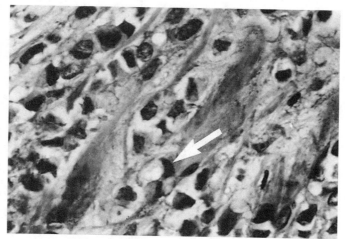

Figure 027 Single-file arrangement of cells with pleomorphic nuclei within a fibrous stroma; presence of a signet ring cell.

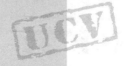
ID/CC   A 68-year-old white woman visits her dermatologist because of a long-standing **itching, painless, scaling, and oozing erythematous rash** over her right **nipple**.

HPI   Her **first menstrual period** started at age 9, and she has **never** been married or **had children**; her **menopause started at age 56**.

PE   **Nipple** on right breast **retracted** and appears **eczematous** with **redness**, some edema, and **desquamation**; **oozing** of yellowish exudate; painless left axillary **lymphadenopathy**; no hepatomegaly or lumps in opposite breast.

Gross Pathology   Ductal carcinoma with extension to overlying skin.

Micro Pathology   Characteristic cells are scattered in the epidermis and are mucin positive and have large nuclei and abundant, pale-staining cytoplasm (PAGET'S CELLS); immunohistochemistry for determining estrogen/progesterone receptor status.

Treatment   Modified radical mastectomy with axillary lymph node dissection; adjuvant tamoxifen therapy when associated ductal carcinoma is estrogen and progesterone receptor positive.

Discussion   Paget's carcinoma is a scaly skin lesion in the **areola and nipple** arising from **ductal adenocarcinoma** within subareolar excretory ducts and progressing outward.

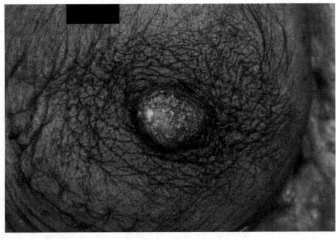

Figure 028 Erosion and crusting of the nipple.

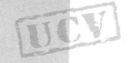

ID/CC	A 52-year-old unmarried white **nulliparous female** smoker with **early menarche** presents with a **painless lump** in her right breast.
HPI	The patient has a **history of atypical hyperplasia** of the right breast. Her **mother died of breast cancer** at 46 years of age.
PE	A 3-cm, **fixed, hard, and nontender mass** in **upper outer quadrant** of right breast; **retraction of overlying skin and nipple**; no nipple discharge; **palpable axillary lymph nodes** on right side.
Labs	Routine lab work normal; normal alkaline phosphatase (no bone metastases).
Imaging	Mammo: **spiculated mass with architectural distortion and multiple clustered pleomorphic microcalcifications**; skin thickening and retraction. CXR: no evidence of metastasis.
Gross Pathology	Hard, irregular whitish mass with granules of calcification and focal yellow areas of necrosis. Profound **fibrosis with induration** in stroma (DESMOPLASTIC REACTION).
Micro Pathology	FNA: large pleomorphic cells arranged in glands, cords, nests, and sheets in dense fibrous stroma; tumor cells **estrogen and progesterone receptor negative** by flow cytometry. Core biopsy: anaplastic cells with high mitotic index consistent with infiltrating ductal adenocarcinoma, not otherwise specified.
Treatment	Surgery; adjuvant chemotherapy; radiation therapy for selected cases; hormonal agents (e.g., tamoxifen) depending on estrogen and progesterone receptor status; rehabilitative measures such as breast reconstruction surgery.
Discussion	Infiltrating ductal breast carcinoma is the **most common type of breast cancer.** Approximately one in nine women in the United States will develop breast cancer. Risk factors include **family history, early menarche, late menopause, obesity, exogenous estrogens, atypical hyperplasia of breast,** and breast cancer in the opposite breast.

GYN

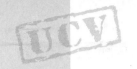

CASE 30

ID/CC	A **25-year-old** black female visits her family doctor for a **painless right breast lump** that she discovered on self-examination; she is otherwise asymptomatic.
HPI	Her medical history is unremarkable.
PE	**Small, encapsulated, well-defined, rubbery, freely movable** 3-cm mass in right lower quadrant of right breast; no overlying skin changes; no nipple retraction; no lymphadenopathy; other breast normal.
Labs	All routine lab work normal.
Imaging	Mammo: oval low-density lesion with smooth margins; "**popcorn calcifications**" seen with degeneration. US: homogeneous, well-circumscribed, hypoechoic mass with visible echogenic capsule.
Gross Pathology	Solid mass; no areas of necrosis or hemorrhage (central myxoid degeneration in older patients).
Micro Pathology	Glandular structures with ductal and stromal proliferation with no cellular atypia.
Treatment	Surgical excision.
Discussion	Fibroadenoma is the **most common benign breast tumor in young women**; it sometimes enlarges during pregnancy or normal menstrual cycles.

Figure 030 Elongating, branching glands with bland proliferative epithelium and loose pale fibrous stroma.

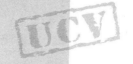

CASE 31

ID/CC   A 22-year-old **female** presents with an **abnormal cervical Pap smear.**

HPI   She has no history of irregular menstrual bleeding, postcoital bleeding, intermenstrual bleeding, or vaginal discharge. She delivered her **first baby at the age of 18** and has had **multiple sexual partners.**

Imaging   Colposcopy reveals a suspicious area from which a biopsy is taken.

Micro Pathology   Biopsy shows loss of normal orientation of squamous cells; atypical cells seen with wrinkled nuclei and perinuclear halos involving full thickness of squamous epithelium; **basement membrane intact.**

Treatment   Local ablative measures such as cryosurgery, laser ablation, or loop excision followed by regular screening surveillance.

Discussion   Cervical dysplasia is a precursor of cervical squamous cell carcinoma; it is associated with **infection with human papillomavirus (HPV) types 16, 18, and 31.**

GYN

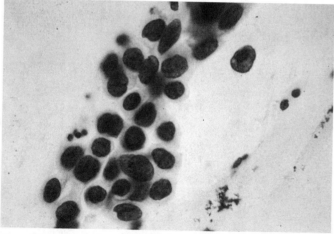

Figure 031 Pap smear showing small cells with hyperchromatic nuclei irregular nuclear contours and scant cytoplasm.

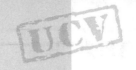

CASE 32

ID/CC   A 29-year-old **Vietnamese female** visits her family doctor because of protracted **nausea, vaginal bleeding, dyspnea, and hemoptysis**.

HPI   Her history reveals one previous normal gestation and one spontaneous abortion as well as a dilatation and curettage 4 months ago for a **hydatidiform mole**.

PE   Vaginal examination with speculum reveals **bluish-red vascular tumor** and **enlarged uterus**; adnexa and ovaries normal.

Labs   **Markedly elevated** serum and urinary **hCG levels**.

Imaging   CXR: **multiple metastatic nodules** ("CANNONBALL" SECONDARY LESIONS).

Micro Pathology   Exaggerated trophoblastic (cytotrophoblastic and syncytiotrophoblastic) tissue proliferation with endometrial penetration; cellular atypia and hematogenous/lymphatic spread.

Treatment   Chemotherapy; follow-up with serial serum hCG levels.

Discussion   Choriocarcinoma is a malignant gestational tumor that may develop during normal pregnancy, after evacuation of hydatidiform mole, or after previous spontaneous abortions.

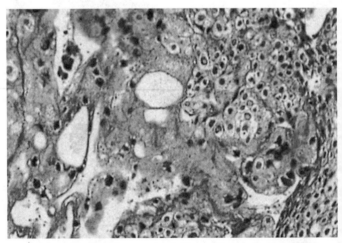

Figure 032 Multinucleated syncytiotrophoblasts with vacuolated cytoplasm adjacent to sheet of smaller mononuclear cytotrophoblasts.

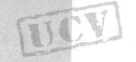

CASE 33

ID/CC
A 33-year-old Hispanic **multigravida** in her 20th week of pregnancy comes to the gynecologist's office complaining of a **mass in her abdomen.**

HPI
She is **pregnant for the fifth time.** She has had no prior abortions or C-sections.

PE
VS: BP normal. PE: no edema; uterus correct height for gestational age (at level of umbilicus); **ill-defined, painless, nonmovable mass** 5 cm from midline on mesogastrium; skin not red or warm; no exudate; no fluctuation; **mass seems to disappear on contraction of rectus muscle.**

Labs
Routine lab work on blood, urine, and stool normal.

Imaging
CT/MR, abdomen: circumscribed mass.

Gross Pathology
Coarsely trabeculated tumor resembling scar tissue; appears to **arise from musculoaponeurotic wall.**

Micro Pathology
Elongated, spindle-shaped cells; fibroblastic process; no evidence of atypical mitoses on biopsy.

Treatment
Wide surgical excision; radiotherapy for recurrent disease.

Discussion
A type of fibromatosis of the anterior abdominal wall in women, desmoid tumor is associated with previous trauma, multiple pregnancies, and Gardner's syndrome. It **frequently recurs after excision.**

GYN

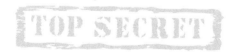

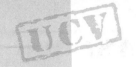

ID/CC A 16-year-old girl is seen with complaints of **colicky lower abdominal pain** together with nausea and vomiting associated with the **onset of menses**.

HPI She achieved menarche at 14, and her initial cycles were irregular but painless (due to anovulation). She does not complain of menstrual irregularity or excessive bleeding and has no urinary complaints or diarrhea.

PE Abdominal exam normal; gynecologic exam reveals blood-stained pad; pelvic exam not performed due to intact hymen; rectal exam normal.

Labs Routine lab parameters normal.

Treatment Symptomatic relief with **prostaglandin synthetase inhibitors** such as mefenamic acid or naproxen sodium; intractable symptoms may require **suppression of ovulation** using combined estrogen/progesterone or progestogens.

Discussion **Primary dysmenorrhea** is defined as **painful periods** for which no organic or psychological cause can be found. Diagnosis is made on the basis of clinical findings. The pain is colicky and usually begins shortly after or at the onset of menses; it is thought to be due to an increase in the production of prostaglandins, leading to uterine vasoconstriction and painful contractions. Occurring **only during ovulatory cycles**, primary dysmenorrhea is most commonly found in women under the age of 20.

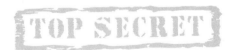

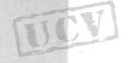

ID/CC
A 60-year-old **obese, nulliparous** white **female** presents with intermittent **postmenopausal vaginal bleeding** of 3 months' duration.

HPI
She has a history of **diabetes, hypertension**, and **infertility with polycystic ovaries; menopause began at 56 years of age.**

PE
Uterus is not enlarged on bimanual palpation.

Labs
CBC: mild anemia. Stool and urine tests within normal limits; endometrial biopsy diagnostic.

Imaging
US, pelvis: **thickening** of **endometrial stripe.**

Micro Pathology
Endometrial biopsy shows endometrioid adenocarcinoma.

Treatment
Radiation therapy; hysterectomy.

Discussion
Endometrial carcinoma is the most common gynecologic malignancy. It is associated with hyperestrogenic states, and depth of myometrial invasion is an important prognostic factor. Postmenopausal bleeding should be considered to be secondary to endometrial cancer until proven otherwise.

GYN

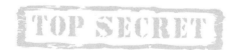

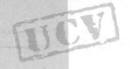

ID/CC
A 27-year-old white female is admitted to the **infertility clinic** for evaluation of her **inability to conceive**; she also complains of **pain during intercourse** (DYSPAREUNIA) and **pain during menses** (DYSMENORRHEA).

HPI
She is **nulligravida**. She admits to having **rectal pain during menstruation**; she also complains of having an **abundant menstrual period** (MENORRHAGIA OR HYPERMENORRHEA).

PE
Bluish spots in posterior fornix on vaginal speculum exam; on bimanual exam, **fixed, tender bilateral ovarian masses palpable during menstruation**; **induration in pouch of Douglas** with **multiple small nodules** palpable through posterior fornix.

Labs
CBC: mild anemia; normal WBC count. ESR normal.

Imaging
Laparoscopy, pelvis: ovaries adhere to broad ligament and show retraction and scarring in addition to **endometriomas**, with dense peritubal and periovarian **adhesions** and **thickening of uterosacral ligaments**; biopsy of suspected lesions is taken. US, pelvis: nonspecific cystic enlargement of ovaries.

Gross Pathology
Brownish nodules on uterosacral ligaments, ovaries, and pouch of Douglas.

Micro Pathology
Laparoscopic biopsy of affected areas shows nodules consisting of endometrial glands, stroma, and hemosiderin pigment.

Treatment
Pain control with NSAIDs or opioids; alter hormonal environment with oral contraceptives, GnRH agonists, or danazol; if medical therapy fails, laparoscopic removal/coagulation of lesions or hysterectomy.

Discussion
Endometriosis refers to endometrial tissue that is present outside the uterus and produces symptoms that vary with location. It is the most common cause of chronic pelvic pain in women. Endometrial implants (endometriomas or "**chocolate cysts**") most frequently involve both **ovaries**.

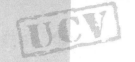

CASE 37

ID/CC
A 42-year-old Filipina in her **20th week of pregnancy** presents with **vaginal bleeding but no pain.**

HPI
She has been feeling inordinately **nauseated** and has suffered from ringing in her ears.

PE
VS: moderate hypertension (BP 150/95). **Uterus large for gestational age** (three finger breadths above umbilicus); lower extremity 2+ **non-pitting edema.**

Labs
Markedly increased β-hCG. UA: **proteinuria** but no casts seen on microscopic exam. Elevated blood uric acid level. Karyotype: diploid XX (complete mole); triploid XXY or XXX (partial mole).

Imaging
US, pelvis: complex "**snowstorm**" **appearance** and **no fetal parts** in uterine cavity.

Gross Pathology
Characteristic appearance of **clusters of grapes.**

Micro Pathology
Chorionic villi markedly enlarged and hydropic with surrounding cyto- and syncytiotrophoblastic tissue proliferation and lack of adequate vascular supply.

Treatment
Dilatation and suction curettage, periodic determination of hCG levels to identify development of invasive mole or choriocarcinoma.

Discussion
A gestational neoplasm that may present as painless vaginal bleeding, **preeclampsia** in the first trimester, or **hyperemesis** gravidarum, hydatidiform mole may develop into **malignant choriocarcinoma** (20%). Hydatidiform mole is more common among females at extremes of reproductive age.

GYN

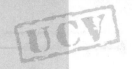

ID/CC   A 53-year-old female complains of **increasing fatigue, insomnia, and depression**.

HPI   For the past 6 months she has had episodes in which her **face and neck have become hot and red** (HOT FLASHES). She has been **amenorrheic for the past 7 months**; prior to this, her menstrual history was normal.

PE   **Thinning of the skin**; **hirsutism**; **atrophic vaginal mucosa** with decreased secretions.

Labs   **Increased 24-hour urinary gonadotropins** (LH and FSH).

Imaging   DEXA: reveals osteoporosis. XR, plain: **osteoporosis** of thoracolumbar spine.

Treatment   Treat osteoporosis with **bisphosphonates, calcitonin**, or selective estrogen receptor modulators; **estrogens** indicated for management of **vasomotor symptoms**.

Discussion   The estrogen deficiency state produced by menopause has short-range (hot flashes), medium-range (vaginal atrophy), and long-range (osteoporosis) consequences that can be relieved or prevented by estrogen replacement. Common side effects in patients taking hormone replacement therapy include irregular bleeding, weight gain, fluid retention, and endometrial hyperplasia. Nevertheless, postmenopausal bleeding should be worked up with an endometrial biopsy to rule out endometrial cancer.

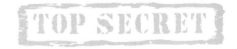

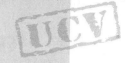

CASE 39

ID/CC	A 56-year-old white nulliparous woman is referred for evaluation of a pelvic mass found on a routine physical.
HPI	She reports increased frequency of micturition and irregular periods until they ceased 3 years ago. She has a history of breast cancer in the distant past.
PE	Large cystic mass the size of a grapefruit in right pelvis that can be felt above the pubis symphysis.
Labs	CA-125 levels elevated; LFTs normal.
Imaging	CT/US, pelvis: cystic pelvic mass arising out of right ovary.
Gross Pathology	Partly solid and partly cystic mass.
Micro Pathology	Papillary structures of neoplastic ciliated columnar cells; psammoma bodies.
Treatment	Surgical staging and resection; chemotherapy.
Discussion	Ovarian cancer is the second most common gynecologic cancer; the serous type is most common and is often bilateral. It is often advanced at the time of diagnosis (omental masses, liver masses, ascites).

GYN

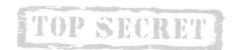

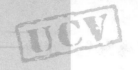

CASE 40

ID/CC	A 20-year-old Asian **female** visits her family doctor because of **chronic, intermittent left lower quadrant pain.**
HPI	The pain is not accompanied by dyspareunia, menstrual irregularity, vaginal discharge, abdominal distention, nausea, vomiting, or diarrhea. It is not correlated with her menstrual periods.
PE	**Left adnexal mass** on bimanual exam; uterosacral ligaments normal; pouch of Douglas normal; McBurney's point nontender; no evidence of ascites.
Labs	Routine lab work on blood, urine, and stool normal; CA-125 levels not elevated.
Imaging	US, pelvis: **large (5-cm) simple cyst in left ovary.**
Micro Pathology	Vaginal smears for cytohormonal evaluation reveal excessive estrogenic stimulation and lack of progestational effect.
Treatment	Follow-up by ultrasound (sizable percentage disappear spontaneously); laparoscopic removal if persistent.
Discussion	Most ovarian cysts are benign. Follicular ovarian cyst is the most common cause of ovarian enlargement.

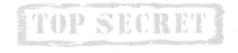

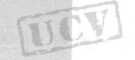
ID/CC   A **25-year-old woman** complains of **loss of weight** and intense right lower abdominal pain and nausea that began when she went jogging yesterday afternoon.

HPI   Intermittent episodes of similar pain have occurred over the past several days. She has regular menstrual cycles with average flow and no dysmenorrhea and had her last period 3 weeks ago.

PE   VS: mild hypotension; normal HR (HR 90). PE: **right lower quadrant tenderness**; pelvic exam reveals tender, mobile 6-cm **right adnexal mass** anterior to uterus.

Labs   CBC: normal; pregnancy test negative.

Imaging   XR, KUB: irregular **calcified** mass in region of right ovary. US, pelvis: **cystic tumor** about 8 cm in diameter replacing the right ovary.

Gross Pathology   Cystic mass replacing the right ovary; thin, **fibrous wall with solid nodule at one aspect containing sebaceous material and matted hair**; tooth structures also seen.

Micro Pathology   Mature tissue elements **representing all three germ cell layers** are present, including skin with adnexal structures, bone, cartilage, teeth, thyroid, bronchi, intestine, and neural tissue.

Treatment   Surgical resection curative.

Discussion   Primary benign teratomas or dermoid cysts originate from germ cells; tumors are cystic and contain elements of all three germ cell layers. Complications of teratomas include torsion, infection, rupture leading to chemical peritonitis, infertility, secretion of thyroid hormone leading to hyperthyroidism (STRUMA OVARII), and carcinoid syndrome due to serotonin secretion; rarely, squamous cell carcinoma may develop in a dermoid cyst.

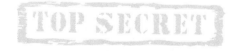

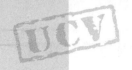

ID/CC A **23-year-old** married **woman** is seen with complaints of **inability to conceive** after a year of unprotected intercourse (INFERTILITY).

HPI Her last menstrual period was 3 months ago, and since menarche she **has only 4 to 5 periods each year** (OLIGOMENORRHEA); a pregnancy test at home was negative. She also complains of **excessive facial hair**. Her **father was diabetic**.

PE Patient **obese**; excessive **facial hair and male-pattern hair distribution on rest of body** (HIRSUTISM) but no virilization; pelvic exam normal; secondary sexual characteristics well developed.

Labs **Elevated LH; decreased FSH** and loss of normal periodicity (LH > FSH, 3:1 ratio); **serum testosterone and androstenedione elevated; serum estradiol** (total and free) within normal limits in early and midfollicular phases; **pattern of secretion abnormal with no preovulatory or mid-luteal increase**; TSH and prolactin levels normal.

Imaging US, transvaginal (high resolution): morphologic features of **polycystic ovaries** (multiple peripheral follicles < 8 mm in diameter; prominent echodense stroma).

Gross Pathology Ovaries enlarged with **pearly-white capsule** and multiple cysts averaging 1 cm in diameter within stroma.

Micro Pathology Cysts **lined by granulosa and theca cells**, the latter luteinized; stroma shows **hyperthecosis** and fibrosis.

Treatment Reduce weight through diet and exercise; ovulation induction with clomiphene; laparoscopic ovarian diathermy or laser drilling in drug-resistant cases; low-dose combined contraceptive pill if contraception is desired.

Discussion Polycystic ovarian syndrome (**Stein–Leventhal syndrome**) is a clinical syndrome of **obesity, hirsutism, and secondary amenorrhea or oligomenorrhea with infertility due to anovulation**, accompanied by multiple-follicle cysts within both ovaries. PCOS patients are at increased risk for breast and endometrial carcinomas (due to unopposed LH stimulation).

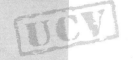

CASE 43

ID/CC   A 17-year-old white **female** visits her family physician because she **has never had a menstrual period** (PRIMARY AMENORRHEA) and **lacks breast development**.

HPI   She has a history of **low birth weight** and lymphedema of the hands and feet.

PE   Short stature; low-set ears; **webbed neck**; cubitus valgus; low hairline; **shield-like chest with widely spaced nipples; harsh systolic murmur heard on back** (due to coarctation of aorta); hypoplastic nails; short fourth metacarpals; high-arched palate; **absence of pubic and axillary hair**; small clitoris and uterus; ovaries not palpable.

Labs   High serum and urine FSH and LH; **no Barr bodies** on buccal smear. Karyotype: 45,XO.

Imaging   US, pelvis: infantile streak ovaries. Echo: bicuspid aortic valve.

Gross Pathology   Fibrotic and atrophic ovaries.

Micro Pathology   Absence of follicles in ovaries; normal ovarian stroma replaced by **fibrous streaks**.

Treatment   Growth hormone and androgens for increase in stature; subsequent estrogen therapy to protect against osteoporosis.

Discussion   The most common karyotype is 45,XO; less common is mosaicism. Turner's syndrome is associated with frequent skeletal, renal (horseshoe kidney), and cardiovascular anomalies (coarctation of the aorta) as well as with hypothyroidism.

GYN

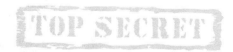

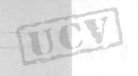

CASE 44

ID/CC   A 39-year-old **black female** presents with a several-month-long history of **profuse menstruation** (HYPERMENORRHEA) **and frequent menstrual periods** (POLYMENORRHEA).

HPI   Further questioning also reveals **painful periods** (DYSMENORRHEA) and increasing **urinary frequency.** She has a history of **infertility and recurrent spontaneous abortions.**

PE   **Enlarged, irregular uterus** on bimanual palpation with several masses on posterior wall.

Labs   CBC/PBS: hypochromic, microcytic anemia.

Imaging   US, pelvis: **multiple heterogeneous masses** distorting uterus.

Gross Pathology   Occur in myometrium (95% are intramural) and are round, firm, and well circumscribed.

Micro Pathology   Interlacing bundles of uniform, differentiated, elongated smooth muscle cells with few mitoses and no anaplasia; malignant transformation rare.

Treatment   Myomectomy; hysterectomy; gonadotropin-releasing hormone analogs.

Discussion   The **most common tumor of the uterus** and the **most common tumor in women,** uterine fibroids are **estrogen-dependent** and commonly occur after 30 years of age; they tend to regress after menopause unless the patient is on hormone replacement therapy.

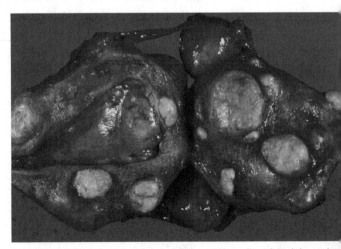

Figure 044 Multiple firm circumscribed, homogenous, yellowish nodules in the myometrium and protruding into endometrial cavity.

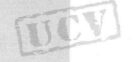
ID/CC	A 60-year-old woman visits her gynecologist because of a **foul-smelling, blood-tinged, purulent vaginal discharge.**
HPI	She has never been married and **has never been pregnant.** She is hypertensive and takes oral hypoglycemic agents for diabetes mellitus.
PE	VS: BP normal at present. PE: overweight; **fleshy, bulky, fungating tumor** protruding from cervical os on vaginal speculum exam.
Imaging	CT/MR: large, complex mass arising from uterus.
Gross Pathology	Large, fleshy tumor of myometrium with areas of necrosis and hemorrhage.
Micro Pathology	Background of spindle-shaped cells with **more than 10 mitoses per high-power field** on biopsy; many mitoses have abnormal mitotic spindle.
Treatment	Adriamycin, progestins, combination chemotherapy. Surgical therapy (total abdominal hysterectomy with bilateral salpingo-oophorectomy, or TAH-BSO) with adjuvant chemotherapy or radiation therapy.
Discussion	A highly aggressive malignant tumor of myometrium, leiomyosarcoma of the uterus may arise in a leiomyoma or de novo. It spreads by contiguity, hematogenously, and through lymphatics.

GYN

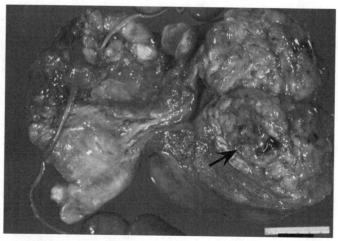

Figure 045 Large fleshy tan mass in the mymetrium with areas of hemorrhage softening and focal necrosis.

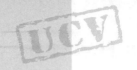

CASE 46

ID/CC A **65-year-old woman** is referred for intractable vulvar growth and **pruritus**.

HPI She has also felt an obstruction in the flow of her urine. She was a **prostitute** and was treated often for STDs. She is a **chronic smoker**.

PE Gynecologic exam reveals excoriation marks over vulva; exophytic growth arising from left labia majora; left inguinal lymphadenopathy.

Labs Cystoscopy reveals lower urethral stenosis (due to involvement by vulvar growth).

Gross Pathology Gross examination reveals firm, exophytic growth.

Micro Pathology Microscopic exam of punch biopsy specimen reveals invasive, well-differentiated **squamous cell carcinoma with keratinization**.

Treatment Confirm diagnosis with biopsy; preoperative radiotherapy to shrink tumor mass; radical vulvectomy with lymph node dissection.

Discussion Vulvar cancer is a disease of **older women** with a mean age of 65 years. It is associated with **smoking**, and its recent increase in incidence among younger women is associated with **papillomavirus**. Carcinoma in situ (vulvar intraepithelial neoplasia, or VIN) and squamous dysplasia are considered precursor lesions. **Cloquet's node** indicates distant metastases.

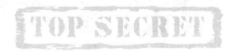

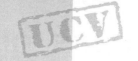

CASE 47

ID/CC A 75-year-old white **woman** visits her gynecologist for a routine checkup and is found to have **white spots** on her **genitalia**.

HPI She complains of slight outer vaginal **itching** but denies any post-menopausal bleeding, vaginal discharge, or drug intake.

PE **Hypochromic macules** on labia majora extending to perineum and inner thighs in patchy distribution with **scale formation** (DESQUAMATION); **skin thickened and rough** (HYPERKERATOTIC); no regional lymphadenopathy; atrophic vaginitis on vaginal speculum exam.

Micro Pathology Biopsy reveals hyperkeratosis and fibrosis with thinning of squamous epithelium; lymphocytic inflammatory infiltration, most prevalent surrounding blood vessels; no chronic inflammatory response; no signs of malignant transformation.

Treatment Biopsy; subsequent treatment dependent on diagnosis. Treat with topical steroids unless malignancy is found.

Discussion **Vulvar leukoplakia** is a clinical diagnosis that can be attributed to a variety of disorders that all produce white patches. Causes may be benign disorders such as vitiligo, as well as inflammatory conditions, premalignant conditions (e.g., dystrophies), or squamous cell carcinoma. **Always perform a biopsy.**

GYN

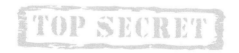

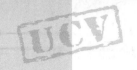

CASE 48

ID/CC	A **73-year-old** woman is brought to a gynecologist by her daughter, who became aware of a **genital ulcer** while helping her mother shower.
HPI	Her history reveals **weight loss** and **dyspnea** together with hypertension and arthritis.
PE	Hard, nodular, 5-mm **pigmented and ulcerated** lesion on upper left **labia minora**; no inguinal lymphadenopathy; scattered crepitant rales on chest auscultation.
Labs	CBC/PBS: slight anemia.
Imaging	CXR: **multiple metastatic nodules**.
Micro Pathology	Biopsy reveals malignant melanoma cells with lymphocytic reaction infiltrating into underlying dermis; cells stain **positive for S100 antigen** and are **negative for mucin**.
Treatment	Surgery with regional lymph node dissection and adjuvant chemotherapy.
Discussion	Vulvar malignant melanoma is the second most common vulvar malignancy (the first is squamous cell carcinoma); metastasis and prognosis depend on the extent of vertical growth.

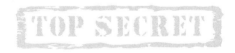

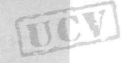

CASE 49

ID/CC	A 25-year-old **woman** presents with **amenorrhea** of 6 weeks' duration and **pelvic pain** over the past day.
HPI	She has a history of **vaginal spotting off and on** for the past 2 weeks and has been using an **IUD** for the past 3 years. She has no history of vaginal discharge and no urinary symptoms, and her previous menstrual history is normal. She has had multiple bouts of **pelvic inflammatory disease**.
PE	VS: BP normal. PE: pallor; abdominal distention and decreased bowel sounds; **cervical motion tenderness**; uterus soft and slightly enlarged on pelvic exam; **soft, tender, boggy mass in right adnexa and pouch of Douglas**.
Labs	CBC: anemia. **hCG levels lower than expected** for this period of gestation; culdocentesis reveals presence of blood in cul-de-sac.
Imaging	US, pelvis: **no products of conception in uterine cavity**; doughnut-shaped mass in right adnexa; echogenic free fluid in cul-de-sac.
Gross Pathology	Extrauterine pregnancy, most commonly tubal.
Micro Pathology	Uterine curettage reveals presence of Arias–Stella reaction in the **absence of villi**.
Treatment	Laparoscopic linear salpingostomy and segmental resection; methotrexate for selected cases without signs of active bleeding or hemoperitoneum.
Discussion	Other risk factors for ectopic pregnancy include **previous tubal surgery**, tubal ligation, **endometriosis**, **previous ectopic pregnancy**, and ovulation induction.

OB

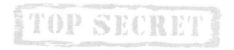

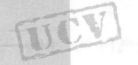

CASE 50

ID/CC   A 38-year-old **grand multipara** develops a marked drop in her blood pressure following **uncontrolled bleeding immediately after delivery**.

HPI   She delivered **twins** at 35 weeks' gestation with **polyhydramnios**.

PE   VS: **hypotension; tachycardia**. PE: anxious; pallor; low central venous pressure; **uterus soft and flabby** with indistinct outline.

Labs   CBC: anemia; mildly decreased hematocrit. Coagulation profile normal.

Gross Pathology   Uterus **grossly overdistended and flabby**.

Treatment   **Fluid resuscitation; blood transfusion; uterine massage**; maintain contraction with an oxytocin infusion; ergotamine for vasoconstriction; if found, **remove retained placenta**; check for cervical, vaginal, or uterine lacerations and uterine rupture; hypogastric artery ligation and/or hysterectomy if other measures fail.

Discussion   Primary postpartum hemorrhage (PPH) is defined as loss of 500 mL or more of blood within 24 hours of a vaginal delivery (1,000 mL after a C-section) or any amount of bleeding that is sufficient to produce a hemodynamic compromise; primary causes include uterine atony, retained placenta, and soft tissue injury. Factors associated with an increased risk of uterine atony and retained placenta include **high multiparity, a maternal age greater than 35 years, delivery after an antepartum hemorrhage, multiple pregnancies, polyhydramnios, a past history of PPH, and coagulation disorders**. Sheehan's syndrome—a clinical syndrome of hypopituitarism secondary to ischemic pituitary necrosis—is a peculiar complication of massive postpartum hemorrhage.

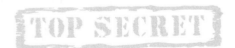

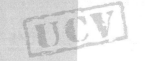

CASE 51

ID/CC
A 28-year-old **woman** presents with **swelling of her entire left leg** of 1 day's duration.

HPI
She delivered a normal full-term male baby 2 days ago.

PE
Left leg **erythematous, warm, swollen,** and **tender.**

Labs
Routine tests normal; normal clotting profile.

Imaging
US, Doppler: clot in left femoral vein. Venography: confirmatory "gold standard" but usually not required.

Treatment
IV heparin and monitoring of clotting time and PTT; elevation of limb; analgesics and soaks.

Discussion
Phlegmasia alba dolens (painful white leg) is due to iliofemoral vein thrombosis occurring in late pregnancy and **postpartum**; it is related to **compression by a gravid uterus** and **hypercoagulability** of pregnancy. Additional risk factors in this population include genetic mutations such as factor V Leiden, smoking, and use of oral contraceptives containing high doses of estrogen.

OB

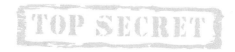

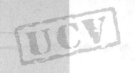

CASE 52

ID/CC	A 30-year-old **woman** presents with fatigue, **significant weight loss**, and **amenorrhea** of 2 years' duration.
HPI	She had a baby 2 years ago and suffered **significant postpartum bleeding**. She bottle-fed her baby because she was **unable to lactate** after delivery.
PE	VS: hypotension (BP 85/60). PE: skin tenting; fine wrinkling around eyes and mouth; loss of axillary and pubic hair.
Labs	**Decreased levels of trophic hormones (FSH, LH, ACTH, TSH, GH, prolactin)**; decreased levels of target gland hormones (T_3, T_4, cortisol, estrogens).
Imaging	MR, pituitary (usually before and after injection of gadolinium DTPA): abnormal signal in pituitary gland.
Gross Pathology	Soft, pale, and hemorrhagic pituitary gland in early stages; shrunken, fibrous, and firm in later stages.
Treatment	Hormone replacement: cortisol; levothyroxine (T_4); estrogen-progesterone replacement.
Discussion	Sheehan's syndrome is most commonly caused by **postpartum infarction of the pituitary**. During pregnancy, the anterior pituitary grows to nearly twice its normal size. During delivery, loss of blood or hypovolemia decreases flow to the pituitary, inducing vasospasm that leads to **ischemic necrosis** of the anterior pituitary. The posterior pituitary is supplied by arteries and is therefore much less susceptible to ischemia. Loss of trophic hormones leads to atrophy of target organs. Ischemic necrosis may also occur in males and in nonpregnant females (trauma, sickle cell anemia, disseminated intravascular coagulation, vascular accidents).

TOP SECRET

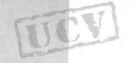
ID/CC   A 30-year-old white **primigravida** at **36 weeks of gestation** visits her obstetrician for the first time in her pregnancy complaining of **swollen legs and headache**.

HPI   Her medical history is unremarkable, and her pregnancy had apparently developed with no complications until the onset of her symptoms.

PE   VS: **hypertension** (BP 170/110). PE: **excessive weight gain** (19 kg); funduscopic exam does not show changes of hypertensive retinopathy; 3+ **pitting pedal edema**; 1+ periorbital edema; fundal height appropriate; fetal parts palpable; fetal heart sounds normal.

Labs   CBC/PBS: complete blood counts and coagulation profile normal. Serum uric acid concentrations raised; mildly elevated AST and ALT; 3+ **proteinuria**.

Imaging   US, OB: single live fetus; lie longitudinal; presentation cephalic; normal biophysical profile; **placental infarctions** seen.

Micro Pathology   Endothelial cell swelling with obliteration of glomerular capillary lumen on renal biopsy.

Treatment   Antihypertensive agents; delivery of fetus and placenta, usually by C-section.

Discussion   Preeclampsia occurs in 5% of all pregnancies; it is most common during the **last trimester of a first pregnancy**. It is characterized by the triad of **hypertension, proteinuria, and edema**. Progression to eclampsia may occur with visual disturbances, seizures, and coma. Other complications include DIC and HELLP syndrome (hemolysis, elevated LFTs, low platelets), which can cause severe liver dysfunction.

OB

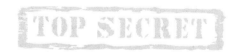

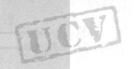

CASE 54

ID/CC   A 5-year-old **Asian** female develops **sudden**, acute **pain** and **loss of vision** in the right eye after watching a series of family slides in a **dark room**.

HPI   She had been complaining of seeing **"halos" around lights** at night.

PE   Injection (due to vasodilation) of ciliary and conjunctival blood vessels; **hazy cornea**; loss of peripheral vision; **markedly elevated intraocular pressure**; shallow anterior chamber with peripheral iridocorneal contact by slit-lamp exam; pupils mid-dilated and unresponsive to light and accommodation; hyperemic and edematous optic nerve bed on funduscopic exam.

Gross Pathology   Pathologically narrow anterior chamber; eye hyperopic and **rock-hard** in consistency; synechia formation; Schlemm's canal may be blocked.

Micro Pathology   Degeneration and fibrosis of trabeculae.

Treatment   Analgesics, IV acetazolamide; topical beta-blockers; steroids; pilocarpine; **laser iridotomy**.

Discussion   Acute angle-closure glaucoma is characterized by a sudden increase in intraocular pressure that may be **precipitated by mydriatics** and upon leaving **dark environments** for well-lit areas.

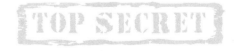

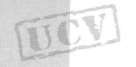

CASE 55

ID/CC

A 28-year-old **woman** presents with a sudden, severe attack of vertigo associated with nausea and vomiting.

HPI

Her symptoms begin and are aggravated when she looks toward the right. The attacks last less than 30 seconds. She has no history of hearing loss, ear discharge, tinnitus, trauma, pain, or restricted neck movement.

PE

Symptoms recur when her head is turned toward right; rotatory fatigable nystagmus with a linear component; no hearing loss or any other neurologic deficit.

Treatment

Reassurance and positioning maneuvers designed to clear debris from the posterior canal.

Discussion

Benign positional vertigo is sometimes seen after head injuries, ear operations, or infections of the middle ear; it is thought to be due to free-floating otoconial debris in the posterior semicircular canal. It typically abates spontaneously after a few weeks or months.

ENT/OPHTALMOLOGY

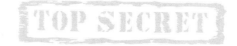

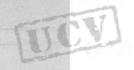

CASE 56

ID/CC   A 35-year-old male seen after a roadside accident presents with a **persistent bloody but thin nasal discharge**.

HPI   Directed questioning reveals that he has also **lost his sense of smell** since the accident.

PE   Watery nasal discharge noted; **bilateral periorbital hematomas** ("black eye") seen; **anosmia** found on neurologic exam; remainder of physical exam normal; on placing a drop of nasal discharge on clean white gauze, **spreading yellow halo noted in addition to central blood stain** ("HALO SIGN"; due to presence of CSF).

Imaging   CT, head: **fracture of cribriform plate**.

Treatment   Antibiotics; head end elevated by 30 degrees; patient **advised not to blow his nose**; neurosurgical consult for possible repair of meninges.

Discussion   Fractures of the base of the skull involve the anterior or middle cranial fossa. Those affecting the anterior fossa, as in this case, may cause nasal bleeding, periorbital hematomas, subconjunctival hemorrhages, CSF rhinorrhea, and cranial nerve injuries (CN I–CN V); **middle cranial fossa structures involving the petrous temporal bone may cause bleeding from the ear, CSF otorrhea, bruising of the ear over the mastoid** ("BATTLE SIGN"), **and cranial nerve injuries** (CN VII–CN VIII).

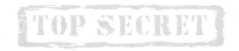

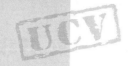

CASE 57

ID/CC   A 50-year-old male complains of hearing loss and a whistling sound in his left ear (TINNITUS).

HPI   He claims to have pronounced **difficulty understanding speech** (out of proportion to hearing loss). He has also experienced occasional **vertigo**.

PE   Left-sided **sensorineural deafness; Weber test lateralized toward right ear**; left-sided corneal reflex lost (CN V dysfunction).

Labs   Pure-tone audiometry reveals sensorineural hearing loss; **discrimination of speech markedly reduced**; loudness recruitment absent; tone decay seen.

Imaging   CT: left **cerebellopontine-angle tumor** suggestive of acoustic neuroma.

Gross Pathology   **Encapsulated tumor** arising out of periphery of CN VIII (vestibular division) at cerebellopontine angle.

Micro Pathology   **Spindle cells** with tightly interlaced pattern (ANTONI A) and **Verocay bodies**.

Treatment   Surgical resection curative.

Discussion   These benign tumors arise from the distal neurilemmal portion of the eighth nerve, usually from the vestibular division, and are correctly called schwannomas; they account for **80% of cerebellopontine tumors**. Acoustic neuromas can be successfully removed, but cranial nerve palsies such as CN VII nerve and deafness are common.

ENT/OPHTALMOLOGY

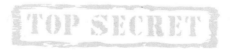

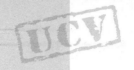

CASE 58

ID/CC
A 30-year-old male complains of sudden-onset **dizziness, nausea, vomiting (nonprojectile), and loss of balance**.

HPI
He also complains of hearing loss and tinnitus. He has **chronic suppurative otitis media** (CSOM) of the right ear, for which he has taken treatment irregularly.

PE
Patient lying on left ear and looking toward right ear; **conductive deafness**; Weber lateralized toward right ear) in right ear; horizontal spontaneous nystagmus toward left; no neurologic deficits.

Imaging
MR, brain and right internal auditory canal: T1-weighted postcontrast images demonstrate enhancing cochlea, vestibule, and semicircular canals on right side. No evidence of brain abscess, neuroma, or cholesteatoma.

Treatment
Antibiotics, vestibular suppressants, and surgical exploration with myringotomy and drainage.

Discussion
Pyogenic inflammation of the labyrinth may result from acute otitis media, operations on the stapes, or preformed pathways such as fracture lines; in CSOM, cholesteatoma may cause erosion of the semicircular canals, exposing the labyrinth to infections. Meningitis is a serious complication of suppurative labyrinthitis.

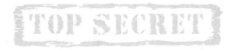

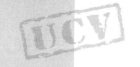

CASE 59

ID/CC   A 45-year-old **obese** man presents with **excessive daytime sleepiness** that has progressively worsened over the past 3 years.

HPI   His wife complains that his **snoring** can be heard in the adjacent room and that he intermittently appears to stop breathing during the night. These **"no-breathing" episodes** last 30 to 90 seconds, and then, with a loud snort, he begins to breathe again. The patient also reports fatigue, forgetfulness, anxiety, **morning headaches**, and diminished sexual interest.

PE   VS: **mild hypertension** (140/90). PE: **short, thick neck; deviated nasal septum; pharyngeal crowding with enlarged, floppy uvula, high-arched palate and soft palate resting on base of tongue.**

Labs   Overnight pulse oximetry reveals **frequent episodes of arterial O$_2$ desaturation; polysomnography** (including EEG, ECG, eye movement, chin movement, air flow, chest and abdominal effort, SaO$_2$, snoring, and leg movement) **diagnostic.**

Treatment   **Weight loss**; avoidance of alcohol and sedatives; **nasal CPAP or BiPAP;** pharmacotherapy with protryptiline; **surgical interventions** include uvulopalatopharyngoplasty (UPPP).

Discussion   Pathophysiologically, nasopharyngeal crowding creates a critical sub-atmospheric pressure during inspiration that overcomes the ability of the airway dilator and abductor muscles to maintain airway patency. This causes apnea, leading to hypoxemia that eventually arouses the patient from sleep. In patients with obstructive sleep apnea, there is an **increased incidence of coronary events, CVAs,** and **right heart failure.**

ENT/OPHTALMOLOGY

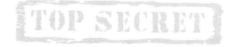

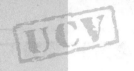

CASE 60

ID/CC A **44-year-old black male** is referred to the ophthalmologist for evaluation of **progressive** and **painless diminution of vision.**

HPI He has no known drug allergies and denies use of steroids.

PE VS: normal. PE: ophthalmology exam reveals normal visual acuity with markedly **reduced peripheral field of vision; elevated intraocular pressure** on tonometry; **increased cup-to-disk ratio with optic atrophy** on ophthalmoscopy; wide open angle noted on gonioscopy.

Treatment **Relief of intraocular hypertension** with topical beta-blockers (timolol), miotics (pilocarpine), or prostaglandin inhibitors with or without surgical procedures such as laser trabeculoplasty, trabeculotomy, goniotomy, and trabeculectomy.

Discussion Open-angle glaucoma is the **most frequent cause** of vision loss in the **African-American population. Risk factors** include **diabetes, nearsightedness,** and **long-term steroid** use. People with **first-degree relatives** with glaucoma are at increased risk. Unfortunately, the disease is usually far advanced when symptoms are first noted. Prevention is through early detection with eye exams once every 2 years or more frequently for those at increased risk.

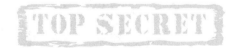

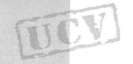

CASE 61

ID/CC

A 60-year-old male complains of progressively diminishing hearing acuity over the past few years.

HPI

The patient's hearing loss is bilateral and is almost the same for both ears; he has no history of ear discharge, tinnitus, or trauma.

PE

Ability to distinguish between consonants markedly impaired; air conduction exceeds bone conduction (due to sensorineural hearing loss); audiometry reveals bilateral hearing loss in higher-frequency range.

Micro Pathology

Presbycusis is characterized by a loss of hair cells, atrophy of the spinal ganglion, altered endolymph production, and thickening of the basilar membrane with some neural degeneration.

Treatment

Hearing aids with high-frequency gain, assistive listening devices, and cochlear implants.

Discussion

Presbycusis is a type of sensorineural hearing loss that results from the aging process; degenerative changes occur in the cells of the organ of Corti and nerve fibers. Deafness is bilateral and symmetrical, commonly affecting the high tones. Other types of presbycusis include strial, which starts in the fourth and sixth decades, is slowly progressive, and is characterized by good discrimination and by the presence of recruitment, a flat or descending audiogram, and patchy atrophy of the middle and apical turns of the stria. Cochlear deafness begins in middle age and is of the conductive variety, showing a downward slope on audiogram and absent pathologic findings. Both types of sensorineural loss can be avoided through use of protection in high-noise areas and monitoring of ototoxic drugs.

ENT/OPHTALMOLOGY

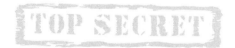

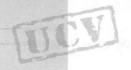
ID/CC A 45-year-old male is seen with complaints of **blurring of vision while reading and performing similar tasks involving near vision.**

HPI He complains that he has to hold the newspaper at an increasing distance in order to read it clearly. He has had no previous problems with his vision and has no history of diabetes or hypertension.

PE **Amplitude of accommodation reduced**; convex lens reduced near-point distance, allowing patient to read comfortably and to engage in tasks requiring near vision.

Treatment Convex lens glasses for work requiring near vision.

Discussion Presbyopia is **natural loss of accommodation** due to **sclerosis of the lens substance**, which fails to adapt itself to a more spherical shape when the zonule is relaxed in the accommodation reflex. Presbyopia is seen in middle-aged patients (mean age 45 years).

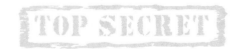

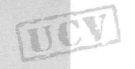

CASE 63

ID/CC   A 29-year-old woman visits a clinic with complaints of **visual blurring**.

HPI   She also complains of **headaches** that are worse in the morning. She has been taking **oral contraceptives** for some time.

PE   VS: BP normal. PE: patient is **obese**; funduscopy reveals presence of **papilledema**; no focal neurologic deficit noted; remainder of exam normal.

Labs   LP: elevated opening pressure; CSF normal.

Imaging   CT: ventricles normal, increased volume of subarachnoid spaces. MR venogram: rules out dural sinus thrombosis.

Treatment   Stop oral contraceptives; advise diuretics and obesity-reducing measures. If medical treatment becomes inadequate, surgical options such as shunt placement are used.

Discussion   Benign intracranial hypertension is primarily a disease of **obese females**; its etiology is unknown, although associations exist with the use of certain drugs (oral contraceptives, steroids, nalidixic acid, tetracycline) as well as with pregnancy, previous head injury, dural sinus thrombosis, and excessive vitamin A intake. Complications include progressive optic neuropathy leading to visual field constriction.

ENT/OPHTALMOLOGY

TOP SECRET

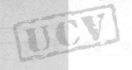

CASE 64

ID/CC
A **16-year-old male** is referred to an ophthalmologist for an evaluation of a **progressively constricting visual field**.

HPI
The boy complains that he sees as though he were looking **through a narrow tube**. Directed questioning reveals that he has a long-standing history of **night blindness** (due to loss of rods). His parents, although normal, had a **consanguineous marriage** and have a **family history of a visual disorder**.

PE
Funduscopy reveals **"bone spicule" pigmentation** in mid-periphery of fundus, waxy appearance of optic disk, and marked narrowing and attenuation of vessels; **field of vision shows concentric contraction** that is especially marked if illumination is reduced.

Labs
Electroretinogram and electro-oculogram demonstrate reduced activity.

Treatment
No satisfactory treatment; genetic counseling for prevention of the disease if the pattern of inheritance in a particular family can be traced.

Discussion
Retinitis pigmentosa is a **slow degenerative disease** of the retina that is always bilateral, begins in childhood, and results in blindness by middle or advanced age; the degeneration primarily affects the rods and the cones, particularly the rods, and commences in a zone near the equator, spreading both anteriorly and posteriorly. The condition may be associated with Laurence–Moon–Biedl syndrome (characterized by obesity, hypogenitalism, and mental subnormality), Refsum's disease (peripheral neuropathy, cerebellar ataxia, deafness, and ichthyosis due to a defect in phytanic acid metabolism), and abetalipoproteinemia. The condition is inherited as an autosomal-recessive trait in 40% of cases, as autosomal-dominant in 20%, and as X-linked in 5%..

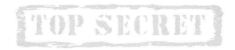

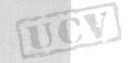

CASE 65

ID/CC	An **18-month-old** boy presents with **diminished visual acuity** and a wandering right eye that his mother noticed while watching him play with his toys.
HPI	On directed history, the child admits to having **eye pain** at night.
PE	**White pupillary or "cat's eye" reflex** in right eye (LEUKOCORIA); deviation of right eye (STRABISMUS); **intraocular mass** on retinal examination.
Imaging	CT/MR, orbit: lobulated, hyperdense retrolental (behind lens) mass; no optic nerve compression.
Gross Pathology	Whitish mass behind lens.
Micro Pathology	Sheets of small, round blue cells with clusters of cuboidal or short columnar cells arranged around a central lumen (FLEXNER–WINTERSTEINER ROSETTES).
Treatment	Surgery; chemotherapy; radiation therapy.
Discussion	The **nonhereditary** variety of retinoblastoma appears as a single tumor; **hereditary** forms occur in early childhood and are often bilateral or multicentric. In hereditary cases, patients are at high risk for other cancers later in life (especially osteosarcoma). Cytogenetic studies reveal a **deletion on chromosome 13** (band 14 on long arm, Rb gene). Rb is a tumor suppressor gene; the loss of both allelic copies leads to malignancy (two-hit hypothesis).

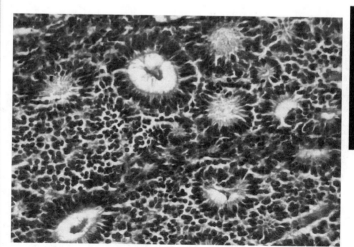

ENT/OPHTALMOLOGY

Figure 065 Diffuse uniform hyperchromatic cells forming rosettes.

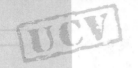

CASE 66

ID/CC   A 30-year-old male presents with sudden-onset **pain, redness, and tearing** in his left eye.

HPI   He also complains of **photophobia and blurred vision** in the left eye.

PE   VS: normal. PE: ophthalmologic exam reveals **conjunctival congestion, diminished visual acuity**, normal visual field, and pupillary miosis with normal reactivity; **aqueous flare with keratic precipitates** noted in anterior chamber on slit-lamp exam.

Labs   CBC: normal. ESR, ANA, RPR, VDRL, Lyme titer (to rule out systemic causes): normal.

Imaging   XR, chest and sacroiliac joints: normal.

Treatment   **Cycloplegics** (atropine) to relax pupillary sphincter and ciliary muscles; **topical corticosteroids**; occasionally immune suppression. Treat **underlying systemic illness**.

Discussion   Systemic disorders (sarcoidosis, SLE, ankylosing spondylitis, tuberculosis, syphilis) should be investigated as causes of uveitis.

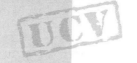
ID/CC

A **5-year-old white** female is brought to her pediatrician because of fever, **marked weakness, pallor, bone pain**, and bleeding from her nose (EPISTAXIS).

HPI

She has a history of progressively increasing fatigability and **recurrent infections** over the past few months.

PE

VS: fever. PE: marked pallor; epistaxis; ecchymotic patches over skin; **sternal tenderness**; slight hepatosplenomegaly with **nontender lymphadenopathy**; no signs of meningitis; normal funduscopic exam.

Labs

CBC/PBS: normocytic, normochromic **anemia; absolute lymphocytosis with excess blasts (> 30%) and neutropenia; thrombocytopenia.** Common acute lymphoblastic leukemia antigen **(CALLA) (CD10) positive**; terminal deoxytransferase **(TDT) positive** (marker of immature T and B lymphocytes) on enzyme marker studies; negative monospot test for Epstein-Barr virus.

Imaging

CXR: no lymphadenopathy.

Gross Pathology

Neoplastic infiltration of lymph nodes, spleen, liver, and bone marrow with loss of normal architecture.

Micro Pathology

Myelophthisic bone marrow (distorted architecture secondary to space-occupying lesions) with lymphoblastic infiltration; lymphoblasts with inconspicuous nucleoli, condensed chromatin, and scant cytoplasm.

Treatment

Treat infection with antibiotics, **anemia** with blood transfusions, and **thrombocytopenia** with platelet concentrations; chemotherapy to induce, consolidate, and maintain remission; intrathecal chemotherapy and irradiation for CNS prophylaxis; bone marrow transplant during remission.

Discussion

Acute lymphocytic leukemia (ALL) is the **most common pediatric neoplasm**; it accounts for 80% of all childhood leukemias. With treatment, it carries a **good prognosis**.

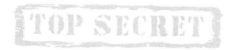

HEM/ONC

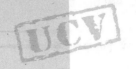

CASE 68

ID/CC	A **25-year-old woman** presents with **high-grade fever, menorrhagia,** and marked weakness.
HPI	Over the past several weeks, she has also had **recurrent infections.**
PE	Marked **pallor**; multiple purpuric patches over skin; hepatosplenomegaly; **gingival hyperplasia**; sternal tenderness; normal funduscopic and neurologic exam.
Labs	CBC/PBS: normocytic, normochromic **anemia**; **thrombocytopenia**; leukocytosis composed mainly of **myeloblasts and promyelocytes** (nonmaturing, early blast cells); **neutropenia**. Prolonged PT and PTT.
Gross Pathology	Bone erosion due to **marrow expansion**; chloroma formation, mainly in skull; splenomegaly.
Micro Pathology	Myeloblasts with myelomonocytic differentiation replace normal marrow (MYELOPHTHISIC BONE MARROW); **basophilic cytoplasmic bodies** (AUER RODS) in myelocytes; **peroxidase-positive** stains on bone marrow and gingival biopsy.
Treatment	Chemotherapy; all-trans retinoic acid in acute promyelocytic leukemia; bone marrow transplant during first remission if HLA-matched donor available.
Discussion	Acute myelogenous leukemia (AML) is not as common in children as is ALL. An increased risk is associated with ionizing radiation, benzene exposure, Down's syndrome, and cytotoxic chemotherapeutic agents.

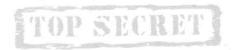

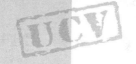

CASE 69

ID/CC
A 12-year-old male presents with high fever, marked **pallor**, and **epistaxis**; he has a history of **recurrent URIs** and high-grade fever that have been treated with parenteral antibiotics.

HPI
He has also shown **marked weakness** over the past 3 months. He lives in the vicinity of an industrial unit that handles petroleum distillates such as **benzene**.

PE
VS: fever. PE: marked pallor of skin and conjunctiva; oral and nasal mucosal **petechiae; purpuric patches** visible on skin; no significant lymphadenopathy; **no hepatosplenomegaly**.

Labs
CBC/PBS: **anemia, neutropenia, and thrombocytopenia** (PANCYTOPENIA); anemia with low reticulocyte count; normal RBC morphology. Normal serum bilirubin; negative Coombs' test; normal chromosomal studies.

Gross Pathology
Increased yellow marrow and decreased red marrow.

Micro Pathology
Hypocellular bone marrow with empty spaces populated by fat cells, fibrous stroma, and scattered lymphocytes; marked decrease in all cell lines.

Treatment
Removal of myelotoxin (in this case, benzene); bone marrow transplantation; immunosuppressive treatment with anti-thymocyte globulin; myeloid growth factors (e.g., GM-CSF) for neutropenia.

Discussion
Sixty-five percent of cases are **idiopathic**. Aplastic anemia following **drug or toxin exposure** may be dose dependent (e.g., benzene, cytotoxic drugs, radiation) or idiosyncratic (e.g., chloramphenicol). Other causes include **viral infection** and Fanconi's anemia, an autosomal-recessive disorder in DNA repair.

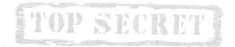

HEM/ONC

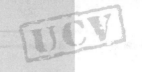
ID/CC   A 66-year-old white man recently **diagnosed with chronic lymphocytic leukemia** comes into the emergency room complaining of **fatigue** and tachycardia.

HPI   He also states that his **urine** has been progressively turning **dark and red** over the course of the day.

PE   VS: tachycardia. PE: dyspnea; pallor of skin and mucous membranes; slight jaundice; **splenomegaly**.

Labs   CBC/PBS: **severe anemia; positive Coombs' test; reticulocytosis;** spherocytosis; "bite cells." UA: positive for hemosiderin. Increased serum indirect bilirubin.

Gross Pathology   Congestive splenomegaly (due to **extravascular hemolysis** in the spleen).

Treatment   Prednisone; transfusions; splenectomy; immunosuppressive drugs. Discontinue any offending drug.

Discussion   Autoimmune hemolytic anemia is idiopathic in about 50% of cases; it is characterized by autoantibodies against RBC membranes (Rh), complement activation, and phagocytosis of RBCs by splenic macrophages. Three main types exist: **warm antibody** (80% to 90%; associated with leukemia, lymphoma, SLE, and viral infections); **cold reacting antibody** (10%; associated with EBV/mycoplasma infections and lymphoma); and **drug-induced** (methyldopa, quinidine, penicillin).

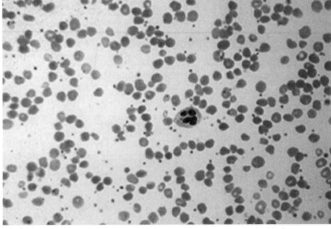

Figure 070 Microspherocytes and polychromasia.

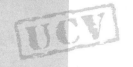

CASE 71

ID/CC   A 35-year-old woman is admitted to the hospital with **left-sided weakness upon awakening**.

HPI   She has **no history** of prior headaches, seizures, hypertension, or diabetes and neither smokes nor takes drugs. Her **first three pregnancies** were **spontaneously aborted**; the fourth resulted in **unexpected fetal death**.

PE   VS: normal. PE: patient conscious; mild pallor; **left hemiplegia** with exaggerated deep tendon reflexes and extensor plantar response (POSITIVE BABINSKI'S SIGN); no neck rigidity; fundus normal; no carotid bruit; no cardiac murmurs; **reddish-blue mottling of skin in fishnet pattern** (LIVEDO RETICULARIS) on extremities; positive Homans' sign in left leg.

Labs   CBC: mild thrombocytopenia. **Prolonged PTT**; normal bleeding and clotting times; **false-positive VDRL** (titer < 1:18); FTA-ABS for syphilis negative; ELISA shows presence of **anticardiolipin antibody (ACA)**.

Imaging   CT, head (24 hours later): hypodensity (due to infarct) in right internal capsule.

Treatment   Initial therapy with heparin followed by warfarin for long-term use; low-molecular-weight heparin may be combined with aspirin for anticoagulation during pregnancy.

Discussion   The presence of **lupus anticoagulant** and ACA defines antiphospholipid syndrome; it is further characterized by **recurrent deep venous thrombosis** in the lower extremities, thrombosis in the renal and hepatic veins, **pulmonary hypertension, cerebral artery occlusion** associated with stroke and transient ischemic attacks (TIAs), and neurologic findings that resemble multi-infarct dementia or epilepsy.

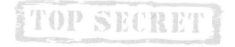

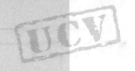

ID/CC   A **9-year-old** girl, the daughter of **African** immigrants, presents with a large **swelling of the left side of her face and jaw** of 3 weeks' duration.

HPI   Two weeks ago, she complained of **loosening of the** upper second left **molar.** Despite the size of the tumor, there is **no pain** associated with it.

PE   Pallor; large, firm, ill-defined **mass** encompassing entire **upper mandible**, producing mild ipsilateral exophthalmos with **deformation** on left side of face.

Labs   CBC/PBS: normocytic, normochromic anemia; mild leukopenia; positive direct Coombs' test. Karyotype: chromosomal translocation t(8;14) involving c-myc gene.

Imaging   CXR: no evidence of mediastinal widening (vs. Hodgkin's lymphoma).

Gross Pathology   Firm, ill-defined tumor involving upper mandible and deforming neighboring structures, but **no ulceration** or necrosis; **no satellite adenopathy.**

Micro Pathology   Giemsa-stained FNA shows cells of uniform size with nongranular basophilic nuclei and some vacuoles, 2 to 5 nucleoli, and evenly distributed chromatin surrounded by small, thin, eccentric cytoplasm that is pyroninophilic; **high mitotic index** and typical "**starry sky**" image pattern (due to diffuse distribution of macrophages among tumor cells).

Treatment   Short-term combination chemotherapy; allopurinol and aggressive hydration with alkalinization to protect against tumor lysis syndrome; alkalinize urine, force diuresis; bone marrow transplantation for recurrent disease; intrathecal methotrexate for meningeal prophylaxis.

Discussion   Burkitt's lymphoma is a small noncleaved lymphoma (**non-Hodgkin's lymphoma**). It is a poorly differentiated **B-cell** lymphoblastic lymphoma. The endemic (African) form is characterized by jaw tumors and is associated with **EBV** infection; the nonendemic (Western) form is characterized by abdominal and pelvic involvement. The condition was first described by Denis Burkitt in 1958 in Uganda.

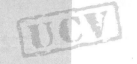

CASE 73

ID/CC
A 65-year-old male visits his family doctor for a routine annual checkup.

HPI
On directed history, he admits to a **weight loss** of about 12 pounds over the past 4 months, together with episodes of **epistaxis** and extreme **fatigue**.

PE
Generalized nontender **lymphadenopathy**; pallor; **enlargement of spleen and liver**.

Labs
CBC/PBS: **markedly elevated WBC count** (124,000); **90% lymphocytes**; no lymphoblasts; mild thrombocytopenia; **Coombs-positive hemolytic anemia; smudge cells** (fragile lymphocytes). CD5 T lymphocytes on flow cytometry.

Imaging
CT/US: hepatosplenomegaly.

Gross Pathology
Lymph node enlargement almost always present; hepatosplenomegaly with tumor nodule formation.

Micro Pathology
Bone marrow biopsy reveals extensive infiltration, mainly by normal-looking lymphocytes and a few lymphoblasts with small, dark, round nuclei and scant cytoplasm; liver, spleen, lymph node involvement common; B lymphocytes fail to mature properly.

Treatment
Chemotherapy; prednisone or splenectomy for complications such as autoimmune hemolytic anemia or immune thrombocytopenia.

Discussion
Chronic lymphocytic leukemia (CLL) is a malignant neoplastic disease of **B lymphocytes** that express the surface marker CD5 (usually in T lymphocytes); it is characterized by **slow progression** of anemia, hemolytic anemia, recurrent infections, lymph node enlargement, and bleeding episodes.

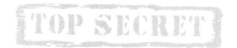

HEM/ONC

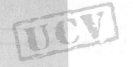

ID/CC	A 40-year-old white male visits a doctor for a life insurance physical examination.
HPI	The patient has no major complaints except for occasional **fatigue** (due to hypermetabolic state) and **increasing abdominal girth** (due to enlarged spleen).
PE	Pallor of skin and mucous membranes; **markedly enlarged spleen; pain on palpation over sternum** (due to marrow overexpansion); no lymphadenopathy; no other abnormalities found.
Labs	CBC/PBS: **markedly elevated WBC count** (130,000); immature granulocytes mixed with normal-appearing ones; **basophilia**; eosinophilia; early thrombocytosis; late thrombocytopenia. **Low leukocyte alkaline phosphatase**; elevated serum vitamin B_{12} level. Karyotype: chromosomal translocation **t(9;22)/bcr-abl gene** (PHILADELPHIA CHROMOSOME).
Imaging	US, abdomen: splenomegaly.
Gross Pathology	Skull chloromas (malignant, green-colored tumor arising from myeloid tissue); enlarged and congested spleen with areas of thrombosis and microinfarcts; hepatomegaly (due to proliferation and infiltration by granulocyte precursors and mature granulocytes).
Micro Pathology	Hepatic sinusoidal leukemic infiltrates; congestive splenomegaly with myeloid metaplasia; Philadelphia chromosome in all myeloid progeny.
Treatment	Imatinib mesylate induces apoptosis via inhibition of tyrosine kinase in cells positive for abr-cbl; hydroxyurea; α-interferon; bone marrow transplantation.
Discussion	In chronic myelogenous leukemia (CML), death usually results from accelerated transformation into acute leukemia (BLAST CRISIS).

TOP SECRET

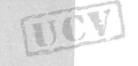
ID/CC

A 55-year-old male presents with **swelling, pain**, and **redness** of the right leg.

HPI

He is retired and leads a **sedentary lifestyle**. He admits to a 70-pack-year smoking history and occasional alcohol intake.

PE

VS: fever (38.4°C); tachycardia (HR 106); mild hypertension (BP 142/92); normal RR. PE: right **lower extremity swollen; pain** elicited on **calf palpation** and on **dorsiflexion** of right foot (HOMANS' SIGN).

Labs

Blood **D-dimer elevated**.

Imaging

US, Doppler: **thrombi occluding right common femoral and popliteal veins**. Venography: **gold standard** for diagnosis, but rarely indicated.

Treatment

Anticoagulation with IV or low-molecular-weight heparin, followed by long-term anticoagulation with oral warfarin or subcutaneous low-molecular-weight heparin.

Discussion

Virchow's triad (**venous stasis, vessel wall injury, and hypercoagulable state**) contributes to the formation of venous thrombi. Complications of DVT include pulmonary embolism and venous ulceration, and insufficiency. Approximately 200,000 deaths per year in the United States are attributable to pulmonary embolism secondary to DVTs.

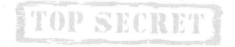

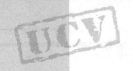

CASE 76

ID/CC	A 25-year-old white female **continues to bleed** steadily after a normal, spontaneous vaginal delivery.
HPI	Manual exploration of the uterus reveals retained placental tissue that requires dilatation and curettage; 30 minutes after the procedure, the patient begins to **bleed profusely from her gums** and continues to bleed vaginally.
PE	Diffuse bleeding in gums and oral mucosa; **bleeding diathesis of skin** (both petechiae and purpura) with **oozing from venipuncture sites**.
Labs	Low fibrinogen. CBC: low platelet count. Prolonged PT and activated PTT; elevated fibrin degradation products, especially D-dimers.
Gross Pathology	May see complications such as renal cortical necrosis, limb thrombosis with gangrene, and ischemic adrenal necrosis.
Micro Pathology	Microthrombi in arterioles and capillaries, leading to **microinfarcts** in practically any organ; also **hemorrhages** and petechiae in involved organs.
Treatment	Treat underlying disorder; fresh frozen plasma; fibrinogen cryoprecipitate; platelets.
Discussion	Disseminated intravascular coagulation (DIC) is a bleeding disorder that is due to consumption of platelets, fibrin, and coagulation factors secondary to excessive clotting in microcirculation. It is precipitated by **cancer, gram-negative septicemia, burns**, multiple **trauma**, and **obstetric complications**.

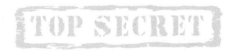

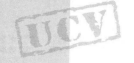

ID/CC
A 35-year-old man complains of **pain in his calf muscles while walking** that is **relieved by rest** (INTERMITTENT CLAUDICATION) together with exertional chest pain.

HPI
He has a family history of **premature atherosclerotic coronary artery disease (CAD).**

PE
VS: mild hypertension. PE: **obese; palmar xanthomas** and tendon xanthomas; **orange-yellow discoloration of palmar creases** (pathognomonic for **dysbetalipoproteinemia**); **tuboeruptive xanthomas** on pressure sites (elbows, buttocks, and knees); weak peripheral pulses.

Labs
LFTs normal; lipid profile reveals **elevated total cholesterol, triglycerides, and VLDL and reduced LDL and HDL**; chylomicron remnants present in fasting plasma; electrophoresis reveals **beta migrating VLDL**; isoelectric focusing shows **EII/EII genotype** (nearly pathognomonic).

Imaging
Angio, coronary: atherosclerotic coronary artery disease confirmed.

Gross Pathology
Yellowish intraluminal atherosclerotic plaques seen in the aorta and other large vessels.

Micro Pathology
Characteristic atherosclerotic plaques.

Treatment
Weight reduction to ideal body weight, regular exercise, **avoidance** of alcohol and other triglyceride-raising drugs; low-fat, low-cholesterol **diet**; fibric acid derivatives and niacin are drugs of choice.

Discussion
Dysbetalipoproteinemia (TYPE III HYPERLIPOPROTEINEMIA) is defined as the presence of **VLDL particles that migrate to the** beta **position on electrophoresis** (normal VLDL particles typically migrate to the pre-beta location). Beta-VLDL particles are chylomicrons and VLDL remnants **caused in part by a mutant apo E** that impairs the hepatic uptake of apoprotein-E-containing lipoproteins (VLDL and chylomicrons).

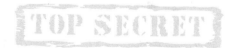

HEM/ONC

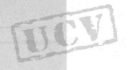

CASE 78

ID/CC	A 61-year-old **white male** presents with marked **weakness, gingival bleeding**, and an **abdominal mass**.
HPI	He has a history of **recurrent bacterial infections** and has not traveled outside the United States.
PE	**Pallor; marked splenomegaly**; mild hepatomegaly; no lymphadenopathy, icterus, or ascites.
Labs	CBC/PBS: **anemia; decreased WBCs and platelets** (PANCYTOPENIA); **lymphocytes with characteristic long, thin cytoplasmic projections** ("HAIRY CELLS").
Imaging	CXR: normal. CT/US, abdomen: massive splenomegaly; mild hepatomegaly; no lymphadenopathy; no evidence of portal hypertension.
Gross Pathology	Liver, spleen, and bone marrow infiltrated by leukemic cells; splenomegaly may be significant.
Micro Pathology	**Bone marrow largely replaced by leukemic cells** (MYELOPHTHISIC BONE MARROW); large proportion are hairy cells and contain tartrate-resistant acid phosphatase (**TRAP**); splenic biopsy reveals leukemic infiltration of red pulp by hairy cells.
Treatment	2-chlorodeoxyadenosine (2-CdA) is first-line therapy; pentostatin, α-interferon, and splenectomy for selected cases.
Discussion	Hairy cell leukemia is a chronic **B-cell** malignancy; autoimmune syndromes are frequently seen, including vasculitis and arthritis. It is also characterized by **atypical mycobacterial infections**.

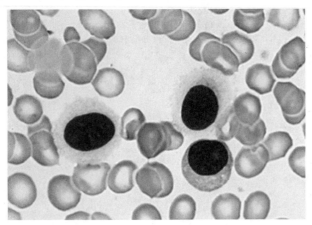

Figure 078 Blood smear with two "hairy" cells and a plasmacytoid lymphocyte. The cytoplasm of the hairy cells is abundant with "hairy" projections.

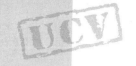

CASE 79

ID/CC An 8-year-old white male presents with an erythematous skin **rash over the buttocks and legs** coupled with **joint pains, abdominal pain**, and **hematuria**.

HPI Three days before he had complained of cough, coryza, low-grade fever, and sore throat. He has a **history of allergy** to dust and pollen.

PE VS: hypertension. PE: **palpable purpuric skin lesions** over buttocks and legs; painful restriction of knee and ankle joint movement with swelling.

Labs CBC: **normal platelet count**; normal coagulation tests. Increased ESR; increased BUN and serum creatinine; elevated antistreptolysin O (ASO). UA: **RBCs and RBC casts** on urinary sediment. Positive stool guaiac test (due to occult blood); elevated serum IgA.

Gross Pathology Necrotizing vasculitis of kidneys and lungs.

Micro Pathology Renal biopsy shows focal and segmental glomerulonephritis with crescents (mesangioproliferative); **mesangial IgA deposits** on immunofluorescence.

Treatment Supportive; steroids; high-dose immunoglobulin therapy experimental; penicillin if ASO titer is elevated.

Discussion Henoch-Schönlein purpura is a generally self-limited, idiopathic disorder that is also known as anaphylactoid or vascular purpura; it is a **common vasculitis** (small vessel) **in children**.

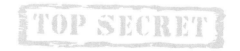

HEM/ONC

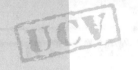

ID/CC	A **6-year-old male** is brought to a specialist by his parents due to persistent **pain and tenderness on the right side of his chest** of a few months' duration.
HPI	There is **no history of trauma** to the affected area. The child is otherwise well and is growing normally.
PE	Exquisitely tender site found overlying fourth rib on right side anteriorly; remainder of exam unremarkable.
Labs	Routine lab parameters normal.
Imaging	CXR: **punched-out lesion** in fourth rib on right side.
Gross Pathology	**Intramedullary expanding, eroding lesion**.
Micro Pathology	Brownish granulation tissue containing **abundant foamy** histiocytes and **eosinophils** with leukocytes and giant cells.
Treatment	Lesions resolve spontaneously; surgical curettage may accelerate healing.
Discussion	Eosinophilic granuloma is a type of Langerhans cell histiocytosis; it is an indolent disorder that affects children and young adults, especially males. Solitary bone lesions may be asymptomatic or may cause pain and tenderness and, in some instances, pathologic fracture, but without any systemic manifestations. Diagnosis is based on radiographic demonstration of a localized destructive lesion arising from inside the marrow cavity. The **skull, mandible**, and **spine** are common locations. In some cases there may be spontaneous healing or fibrosis within a period of 1 to 2 years. The disease may also be multifocal, involving the lung, liver, spleen, or other organs.

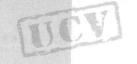

ID/CC   A 2-year-old boy is brought in for a pediatric consultation because his parents are concerned about **the child's protruding eyes** (EXOPHTHALMOS) and **excessive urine volume** (POLYURIA).

HPI   The parents also state that the child has been febrile and has had multiple ear infections.

PE   Low weight for age; bilateral exophthalmos; **painful swellings over head** (due to cystic bony lesions); no icterus; mild hepatosplenomegaly.

Labs   CBC: normal blood counts. **Increased serum osmolality; decreased urine osmolality.**

Imaging   XR, skull: **multiple rounded lytic lesions.**

Micro Pathology   Bone biopsy from skull lesions show granulomatous lesions and characteristic Langerhans cells with coffee-bean-shaped nuclei and pale, abundant cytoplasm; **tennis-racket-shaped tubular structures** (BIRBECK GRANULES) on electron microscopy; positive S-100 protein and CD1 antigen.

Treatment   Combination chemotherapy, curettage of bony lesions.

Discussion   A type of **Langerhan's cell histiocytosis**, Hand–Schüller–Christian syndrome is multifocal, producing **diabetes insipidus** due to the involvement of the hypothalamus and exophthalmos from orbital infiltration by histiocytes.

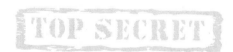

HEM/ONC

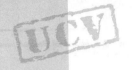

ID/CC A **2-year-old** white male child is seen with complaints of **fever** followed by a **diffuse skin rash**.

HPI The child was apparently well a month ago, born after an uncomplicated pregnancy and delivery.

PE VS: tachycardia; fever. PE: mild pallor; otoscopy of left ear reveals dull, poorly mobile tympanic membrane with pus behind it (OTITIS MEDIA); generalized lymphadenopathy; hepatosplenomegaly; diffuse maculopapular eczematous rash.

Labs CBC: anemia; thrombocytopenia with leukopenia (PANCYTOPENIA); relative eosinophilia.

Imaging CT, abdomen: hepatosplenomegaly. XR: **cystic, rarefied lesions on skull and pelvis**.

Gross Pathology Skin shows presence of extensive **eczematoid rash**; large destructive bone lesions found on skull and pelvis.

Micro Pathology **Eosinophilic granulomatous lesions** in all involved organs; EM shows typical **Langerhans cells with characteristic Birbeck granules**; these cells were further found to be HLA-DR-positive and expressing **CD1 antigen**.

Treatment Corticosteroids; chemotherapy; surgery or radiotherapy for localized bone disease.

Discussion Letterer–Siwe disease is an acute or subacute clinical syndrome of unknown etiology affecting children less than 3 years old. It is marked by fever due to localized infection followed by a diffuse maculopapular eczematous purpuric skin rash and subsequent hepatosplenomegaly and generalized lymphadenopathy. It shows similarities to acute leukemia and other infectious processes. Diabetes insipidus, exophthalmos, and bone lesions are usually seen in combination.

TOP SECRET

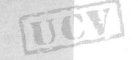

CASE 83

ID/CC	A **24-year-old** white **male** complains of rapid enlargement of his abdomen, producing a dragging sensation, along with a **painless lump in his neck** for the past 2 months.
HPI	The patient also complains of intermittent **fever**, drenching **night sweats**, pruritus, and **significant weight loss**.
PE	Pallor; **unilateral nontender, rubbery, enlarged cervical lymph nodes**; **splenomegaly**; no enlargement of tonsils.
Labs	CBC/PBS: neutrophilic leukocytosis with lymphopenia; normocytic anemia. Elevated ESR and LDH; elevated serum copper and ferritin; negative Mantoux test.
Imaging	CXR: **bilateral hilar lymphadenopathy**. CT, chest: mediastinal lymphadenopathy. CT, abdomen: **splenomegaly, enlarged lymph nodes**, mild hepatomegaly.
Gross Pathology	Involved lymph nodes are rubbery and have **"cut-potato"** appearance of cut surface.
Micro Pathology	Lymph node biopsy shows large histiocyte cells with multilobed nuclei and eosinophilic nucleolus resembling **owl's eyes** (REED-STERNBERG CELLS); no bone marrow involvement on bone marrow biopsy.
Treatment	Radiotherapy and chemotherapy.
Discussion	Four patterns of Hodgkin's disease are seen on lymph node biopsy: lymphocytic predominance 5% to 10%; nodular sclerosis 65% to 75% (seen frequently in young women); mixed cellularity 20% to 30%; and lymphocyte depleted 10%. Prognosis worsens in this order. **Ann Arbor staging** I–IV with subclassification A (no constitutional symptoms) and B (weight loss, fever, night sweats) most accurately predicts prognosis. The disease **spreads to contiguous lymph nodes** before hematogenous dissemination.

TOP SECRET

HEM/ONC

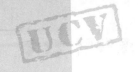

CASE 84

ID/CC   A 3-year-old white female is brought to the emergency room with a skin rash and **severe epistaxis**.

HPI   The patient had a **URI** consisting of a severe cough and a runny nose 10 days **before the onset of her symptoms**. She has no prior history of **prolonged bleeding** following minimal trauma.

PE   **Mucosal petechiae**; epistaxis; **hemorrhagic bullae** in buccal mucosa; extensive purpuric skin rash; spleen nonpalpable.

Labs   CBC: mild anemia; **low platelet count** (10,000); **RBCs and WBCs normal**. Prolonged bleeding time; normal PTT; normal PT; antiplatelet antibodies detected in serum.

Gross Pathology Purpura (due to extravasation of blood from intravascular space into skin); pin-sized hemorrhages (PETECHIAE); ecchymosis (larger than purpura).

Micro Pathology Normal bone marrow aspirate with **increased number of megakaryo- cytes**.

Treatment Prednisone; splenectomy; IVIG.

Discussion Idiopathic thrombocytopenic purpura (ITP) is an **autoimmune disease** with formation of **IgG antiplatelet antibodies** and subsequent platelet destruction in the spleen. It often **follows a viral infection** and is self-limited in children but chronic in adults.

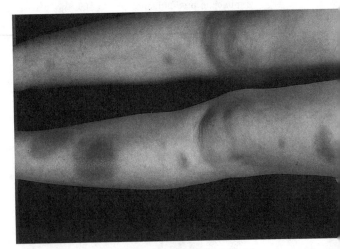

Figure 084 Eccymoses of the lower extremities.

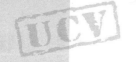

CASE 85

ID/CC   A 64-year-old **black** male suffers from **bone pain**, weight loss, and **easy fatigability**.

HPI   He also complains of **recurrent URIs** and frequent nosebleeds.

PE   Pallor; **bone tenderness** in lower back and ribs; petechiae on buccal mucosa; no hepatosplenomegaly.

Labs   CBC/PBS: **normocytic, normochromic anemia**; neutropenia; **rouleau formation** (RBCs adhering together like stack of poker chips). **Elevated serum calcium**; normal alkaline phosphatase; markedly **increased ESR**; **gamma spike on serum protein electrophoresis** (**monoclonal** gammopathy). UA: **Bence Jones proteinuria** (due to IgG light chains).

Imaging   XR, plain: **punched-out, lytic bone lesions** in vertebrae, long bones, and skull (axial skeleton).

Gross Pathology   Multifocal replacement of normal bone tissue with tumor cells (plasmacytoma); pelvis, skull, and spine most affected.

Micro Pathology   Infiltration of bone marrow by normal-looking plasma cells (abundant cytoplasm, eccentric nuclei) in aggregates; **amyloid deposits** in kidney with renal tubular cast formation and interstitial fibrosis (can cause **renal insufficiency**); bone erosion and destruction of cortical bone.

Treatment   Chemotherapeutic regimen; hydration; treat hypercalcemia and hyperuricemia; consider palliative radiation therapy; allogeneic bone marrow transplantation in selected cases.

Discussion   Multiple myeloma is a **primary malignancy of plasma cells** with replacement of normal bone marrow; it is the most common primary bone cancer. The prognosis worsens with anemia, renal failure, and multiple lytic lesions.

TOP SECRET

HEM/ONC

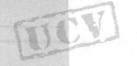

CASE 86

ID/CC A 54-year-old white male complains of **easy fatigability**, shortness of breath, headache, and lightheadedness over the course of almost one year, with increasing severity.

HPI He has also noticed a feeling of heaviness in his abdomen and **increasing girth** as well as recurrent deep pain in the legs and occasionally in the upper abdomen.

PE **Massive splenomegaly**; enlarged liver; moderate amount of ascitic fluid; multiple petechiae on thorax and extremities; **no lymphadenopathy** (one differential feature shared with chronic myelogenous leukemia).

Labs CBC/PBS: anemia (Hb 7.2); **low hematocrit**; anemia; immature WBCs and normoblasts seen simultaneously (LEUKOERYTHROBLASTIC SMEAR); **teardrop-shaped RBCs**; giant abnormal platelets.

Imaging XR, plain: dense bones (generalized osteosclerosis).

Gross Pathology Extramedullary hematopoiesis, which is prominent in liver and spleen, with significant increase in size and weight together with firm consistency.

Micro Pathology "Dry tap" on **bone marrow** biopsy; hypocellular bone marrow (hypercellular early in disease); significant increase in number of megakaryocytes; replacement of marrow tissue with fibrosis (positive reticulin or silver stain); preservation of normal architecture of spleen.

Treatment Transfusions; androgens; α-interferon; splenectomy; allogeneic bone marrow transplantation in younger patients.

Discussion Also called agnogenic myeloid metaplasia, myelofibrosis with myeloid metaplasia is an idiopathic condition in which increased secretion of platelet-derived growth factor (PDGF) and TGF-β causes **replacement of bone marrow tissue with fibrosis**.

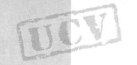

CASE 87

ID/CC	A 53-year-old white male notices **painless lumps** bilaterally **in his neck** that have slowly enlarged over the past 3 months.
HPI	Although he denies any pain, he admits to having episodes of mild **fever**, **night sweats**, and some **weight loss** over this period.
PE	Bilateral cervical **firm lymphadenopathy**; pallor; splenomegaly.
Labs	CBC: Coombs-positive hemolytic **anemia**; thrombocytopenia. **Elevated serum LDH** (a useful prognostic marker); hypogammaglobulinemia.
Imaging	CT/US: lymphadenopathy; splenomegaly.
Gross Pathology	Lymph nodes have grayish hue on outside and **"cut-potato"** appearance of cut surface.
Micro Pathology	Lymph node biopsy demonstrates nodular (well-differentiated) or diffuse-type (poorly differentiated) lymphocytic lymphoma; histiocytic and stem cell lymphoma.
Treatment	Alkylating agents in various combinations; radiotherapy if localized; bone marrow transplantation.
Discussion	Primary malignant neoplasms of lymphocytes arise in lymphoid tissue anywhere in the body; they occur mainly in lymph nodes but may involve intra-abdominal organs and bone marrow. The prognosis is more dependent on grade than on stage. Follicular (B-cell) lymphomas are the most common form and are associated with t(14;18) of bcl-2 (an anti-apoptosis protein). HIV patients have a higher incidence of non-Hodgkin's lymphoma.

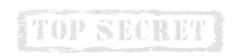

HEM/ONC

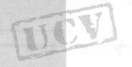

CASE 88

ID/CC
A 62-year-old Jewish **male** visits his family doctor because of **epistaxis**, headache, and dizziness.

HPI
The patient had **black, tarry stools** (MELENA) 2 months ago and was previously admitted to the hospital for **deep venous thrombosis**. He also describes episodes of severe generalized **itching** (PRURITUS), primarily after showering.

PE
VS: **hypertension** (BP 170/100). PE: obese and **plethoric**; mild cyanosis; engorged, tortuous retinal veins with dark red hue on funduscopy; **palpable spleen**.

Labs
CBC/PBS: **markedly increased RBC count, hemoglobin level, and hematocrit**; WBCs and platelets also increased; RBC morphology normal. Normal P_{O_2}, P_{CO_2}, and PT; increased vitamin B_{12} levels; increased leukocyte alkaline phosphatase; increased serum and urine uric acid levels; **decreased erythropoietin level** (distinguishes polycythemia vera from secondary polycythemia).

Gross Pathology
Increased blood volume and viscosity (RBC **sludging** and thrombus formation mainly in heart and brain); subnormal platelet function (bleeding tendency); increased frequency of peptic ulceration.

Micro Pathology
Bone marrow biopsy shows **increase in erythroid series precursors** and, to a lesser extent, in megakaryocytes and WBC precursors; thrombus formation with microinfarcts in brain and heart; myelofibrosis may ensue with characteristic findings.

Treatment
Phlebotomy; hydroxyurea; treat hyperuricemia; splenectomy in selected cases.

Discussion
Polycythemia is characterized by an increase in RBC mass with increased blood volume and viscosity; it may be primary (polycythemia vera) or secondary (due to COPD, smoking, obesity, etc.). PCV may progress to chronic myelogenous leukemia, myelofibrosis, or acute myelogenous leukemia.

TOP SECRET

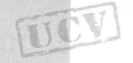

CASE 89

ID/CC
A 4-year-old female is brought by her mother to the pediatric clinic after she finds **blood and a "lump" in the child's vagina**.

HPI
The child's father died of brain cancer, and her mother is receiving treatment for breast cancer. Her grandfather died of metastatic colorectal cancer.

PE
Pelvic exam reveals **ulcerated, polypoid, grape-like mass** arising from wall of vagina.

Labs
Routine lab work on urine, blood, and stool yields no pathologic findings.

Gross Pathology
Bulky tumor mass with multilobed papillary projections resembling mass of grapes.

Micro Pathology
Biopsy of tumor mass shows **desmin- and myoglobin-positive** (muscle tumor), elongated rhabdomyoblasts with large eosinophilic cytoplasm and **cross-striations**.

Treatment
Surgical resection with adjuvant chemotherapy, radiotherapy.

Discussion
Sarcoma botryoides is a polypoidal subtype of **embryonal rhabdomyosarcoma** that characteristically protrudes like a mass of grapes from the vagina or bladder; it is the most common sarcoma in children. Rhabdomyosarcomas are often found in **"cancer families"** (e.g., Li–Fraumeni syndrome).

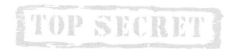

HEM/ONC

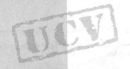
ID/CC A 10-year-old black child presents with a chronic nonhealing ulcer on his lower leg.

HPI He has had recurrent episodes of abdominal and chest pain (due to microvascular occlusion) along with diminution of vision. His maternal cousin suffers from a blood disorder.

PE VS: fever. PS: pallor; mild icterus; funduscopy reveals hypoxic spots with neovascularization ("SEA FANS"); nonhealing chronic ulcer on left lower leg.

Labs CBC/PBS: decreased hematocrit; megaloblastic anemia; sickle-shaped RBCs; Howell–Jolly bodies and Cabot rings; sickling of RBCs on sodium metabisulfite peripheral film (Sickledex prep). Serum bilirubin moderately elevated; quantitative hemoglobin electrophoresis shows 85% HbS. UA: microscopic hematuria.

Imaging CT/US, abdomen: small, calcified spleen.

Treatment Local therapy for leg ulcer; laser therapy for proliferative retinopathy; antibiotic prophylaxis against capsulated bacteria; folic acid supplementation; hydroxyurea may help increase fetal hemoglobin levels; bone marrow transplantation.

Discussion Sickle cell anemia is caused by a point mutation on the gene coding for the β chain of hemoglobin; it shows autosomal-recessive inheritance. Glutamic acid is substituted by valine at position 6, leading to chronic hemolytic anemia. In the reduced form, HbS forms polymers that damage the RBC membrane. Factors that hasten sickling include acidosis and hypoxemia. Prenatal diagnosis is available for at-risk fetuses.

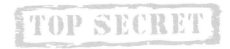

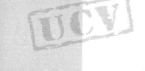

CASE 91

ID/CC   An 11-month-old male presents with marked **pallor, failure to thrive, and delayed developmental motor milestones.**

HPI   The child's parents are **Indian** immigrants.

PE   Marked pallor; mild icterus; frontal bossing and **maxillary hypertrophy** ("CHIPMUNK FACIES"); **splenomegaly.**

Labs   CBC: severe microcytic, hypochromic anemia with **anisopoikilocytosis**; decreased reticulocytosis. **HbA absent; HbF 95%**; mildly increased unconjugated bilirubin.

Imaging   XR, skull (lateral): maxillary overgrowth and widening of diploic spaces with **"hair on end" appearance** of frontal bone, caused by vertical trabeculae.

Gross Pathology   Expansion of hematopoietic bone marrow, causing thinning of cortical bone or new bone formation.

Micro Pathology   Red marrow increased; yellow marrow decreased; marked erythroid hyperplasia in marrow (ineffective erythropoiesis).

Treatment   **Blood transfusion, folic acid supplement, iron chelation therapy** with desferrioxamine to reverse hemosiderosis, splenectomy, and **bone marrow transplantation** using HLA-matched sibling donors.

Discussion   Beta-thalassemia results from decreased synthesis of β-globin chains due to errors in the transcription, splicing or translation of mRNA. Alpha-thalassemia results from decreased synthesis of α-globin chains due to deletion of one or more of the four α genes that are normally present.

HEM/ONC

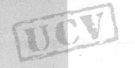

CASE 92

ID/CC   A 23-year-old white **female** diagnosed 2 years ago as **HIV positive** is brought to the emergency room by her husband because of tachycardia, shortness of breath, headache, **intermittent disorientation**, and aphasia.

HPI   She had started prophylactic **TMP-SMX** 3 weeks ago. On the previous day, she had finished her menstrual period, which was abundant and had lasted for 7 days. Her husband also points out a **generalized red rash** all over her body.

PE   VS: tachycardia; **fever**. PE: pale skin and mucous membranes; **confusion** and apathy **with lucid periods**; petechiae on chest and extremities; positive Babinski's sign.

Labs   CBC/PBS: **microangiopathic hemolytic anemia** (Hb 7.2) with striking **reticulocytosis** and **fragmented RBCs** (SCHISTOCYTES); **low platelet count** (50,000); negative Coombs' test. Elevated indirect bilirubin (3.5). UA: hemosiderin and hemoglobin detected. **Absent haptoglobin** (due to intravascular hemolysis); **normal coagulation tests; elevated LDH.**

Gross Pathology   Thrombus formation in several organs with platelet depletion and microangiopathic hemolytic anemia; kidney, brain, and heart most affected by thrombosis.

Micro Pathology   Multiple hyaline thrombi in brain, myocardium, renal cortex, adrenals, and pancreas.

Treatment   Plasmapheresis and fresh frozen plasma exchange; prednisone; splenectomy.

Discussion   Also known as Moschcowitz's syndrome, thrombotic thrombocytopenic purpura (TTP) is an idiopathic disease found in **pregnant** and **HIV positive** patients and following exposure to drugs such as **antibiotics** and **estrogens**.

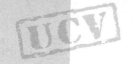

CASE 93

ID/CC   An 18-year-old hospitalized male complains of **fever, nausea, vomiting,** and chest pain following a blood transfusion.

HPI   He was involved in a motorcycle accident and was rushed to the emergency room, where he **received five units of blood** before being taken to the OR for repair of a ruptured spleen and liver.

PE   VS: fever. PS: no hepatosplenomegaly or lymphadenopathy; surgical laparotomy wound unremarkable.

Labs   **Positive Coombs' test** (indicating autoantibodies to RBCs); decreased serum haptoglobin; elevated indirect bilirubin; **cola-colored urine** (due to hemoglobinuria).

Treatment   Hydration; force diuresis with mannitol or furosemide; hydrocortisone; alkalinize urine with HCO_3.

Discussion   Acute hemolytic transfusion reaction may be the result of complete complement activation; most commonly it is a result of **mismatched blood,** producing **intravascular hemolysis**. If severe, renal shutdown or disseminated intravascular coagulation (DIC) may occur.

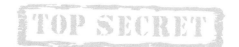

HEM/ONC

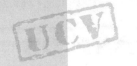

CASE 94

ID/CC
During the administration of a blood transfusion, a 45-year-old male presents with **fever, headache, and facial flushing.**

HPI
An hour later he develops **frank rigors.** He has received **several transfusions in the past,** all of which were uneventful. The last one was **a few weeks ago.**

PE
VS: fever; BP normal; tachycardia. PE: marked pallor; facial flushing; no cyanosis, icterus, or respiratory distress evident.

Labs
CBC/PBS: **negative direct and indirect Coombs' test.** Normal serum bilirubin; no incompatibility found on repeat cross-matching of donor serum and patient's blood.

Treatment
Supportive; antipyretics; **leukocyte-deplete future transfusions** by filtration.

Discussion
Febrile nonhemolytic transfusion reaction is caused by **preformed leukoagglutinins** (cytotoxic antibodies) developed after previous transfusions; it is primarily a **type II hypersensitivity reaction.** Skin rash and pruritus or anaphylaxis occur in allergic reactions mediated by IgE (due to a **type I hypersensitivity reaction**).

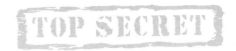

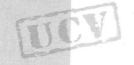

CASE 95

ID/CC
A 12-year-old white female is brought to the emergency room because of **uncontrollable bleeding following a tooth extraction.**

HPI
She has a **history of prolonged bleeding** following minimal trauma. Her **father** also has a **bleeding disorder.**

PE
Mucosal petechiae; epistaxis.

Labs
Prolonged bleeding time; normal platelet count; moderately **prolonged PTT; normal PT; quantitative assay for factor VIII reduced;** subnormal platelet aggregation in response to ristocetin; low von Willebrand's factor (vWF) antigen levels; low vWF activity.

Treatment
Desmopressin, virally attenuated vWF concentrate (Humate-P); avoid aspirin.

Discussion
A common congenital disorder of hemostasis, von Willebrand's disease is also called vascular hemophilia. Types I and II are **autosomal dominant;** vWF factor is necessary for platelet adhesion.

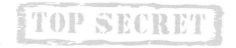

HEM/ONC

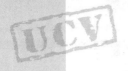

ID/CC
A **68-year-old** white male visits his doctor complaining of **weight loss**, increasing **fatigue**, **weakness**, headache, and **visual disturbances** over the past several months.

HPI
He also complains of **easy bruising** and **bleeding gums** while brushing his teeth.

PE
Generalized **lymphadenopathy**; **engorgement of retinal veins** with hemorrhages; moderate hepatosplenomegaly.

Labs
CBC/PBS: **anemia** (Hb 7.3); RBC **rouleau formation**. **IgM paraprotein** (monoclonal spike on serum protein electrophoresis); increased serum viscosity. UA: normal.

Imaging
XR, plain: **absence of lytic lesions** (vs. multiple myeloma).

Micro Pathology
Lymph node biopsy may be labeled pleomorphic lymphoma; bone marrow and spleen typically infiltrated with plasma cell precursors (plasmacytic lymphocytes); may show cytoplasmic eosinophilic, PAS-positive inclusion bodies (DUTCHER BODIES).

Treatment
Plasmapheresis; chlorambucil; cyclophosphamide; cladribine; autologous stem cell transplantation.

Discussion
Waldenström's macroglobulinemia is a malignant B-lymphocyte disorder characterized by **excessive IgM** (macroglobulin) **production** and **hyperviscosity syndrome**.

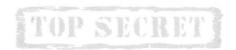

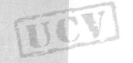

ID/CC

A 2-year-old **male** is brought to his pediatrician because of recurrent **epistaxis** and chronic **eczematous dermatitis**.

HPI

He has a history of **recurring pneumonia** and bilateral **chronic** suppurative **otitis media**. A **male cousin** suffers from a **similar illness**.

PE

Epistaxis; eczematous dermatitis over both legs; several **purpuric patches** over skin; mild splenomegaly and cervical lymphadenopathy.

Labs

CBC/PBS: **thrombocytopenia**; lymphopenia. Decreased isohemagglutinins; decreased IgM; increased IgE, normal IgG, and increased IgA; **inability to form IgM antibody to carbohydrate antigens** (i.e., capsular polysaccharides of bacteria).

Treatment

Largely supportive; intravenous immunoglobulin (IVIG); bone marrow transplant; splenectomy.

Discussion

Wiskott–Aldrich syndrome is a rare **X-linked recessive** disease with **B- and T-cell deficiency** characterized by a **triad of thrombocytopenia, eczema, and recurrent pyogenic infections**; it is due to a deletion of the WASP gene in the p11 region of the X chromosome. The condition is associated with an increased incidence of **lymphomas**.

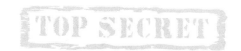

HEM/ONC

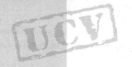

CASE 98

ID/CC	A newborn girl is brought into the genetics department for a karyotype study.
HPI	She was born of a **45-year-old mother** who feels that her child is **developmentally retarded** with **characteristic "mongoloid" facial features**; her pregnancy was uneventful.
PE	Generalized **hypotonia**; flattened face and low-set ears; **macroglossia**; flattened nasal bridge and **epicanthal folds**; silver-white spots on the periphery of irises (BRUSHFIELD SPOTS); single **transverse palmar crease** (SIMIAN CREASE); widely split fixed S2 (due to an atrial septal defect).
Labs	Karyotype: 47,XX; trisomy 21.
Imaging	KUB: **double bubble** (dilated stomach and proximal duodenum) due to **duodenal atresia**. XR, plain: hypoplastic middle and terminal phalanges of fifth digits (ACROMICRIA). Echo: endocardial cushion defect.
Gross Pathology	Brachycephalic head; small brain with shallow sulci; hypoplasia of frontal sinuses; endocardial cushion defect.
Treatment	Surgery for congenital heart defects and duodenal atresia; training in specialized groups.
Discussion	The **most common chromosomal disorder**, Down's syndrome is most frequently caused by trisomy 21 (due to nondisjunction); it is less commonly caused by mosaicism or a Robertsonian translocation. It is associated with a higher incidence with **advanced maternal age** (indication for prenatal screening); a higher incidence of cardiac defects, especially **endocardial cushion defects**; and a higher incidence of **acute leukemia** and **presenile dementia of Alzheimer's type**.

TOP SECRET

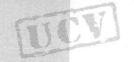

CASE 99

ID/CC
A 7-year-old boy is brought to the optometrist for **diminished visual acuity** and requests a prescription for eyeglasses.

HPI
The boy has an unusual body habitus with long arms and legs; a family history reveals similar body proportions in other family members. He is referred to his family doctor, who on careful questioning discloses that an **uncle died** of a **ruptured aortic aneurysm.**

PE
Tall; **long extremities**; arm span greater than height (DOLICHOSTENOMELIA); **long, slender fingers** (ARACHNODACTYLY); **dislocation of lenses** (ECTOPIA LENTIS); severe myopia; inguinal hernia; high-arched palate; flat feet (PES PLANUS); **aortic diastolic murmur** (aortic insufficiency); funnel chest due to pectus excavatum; scoliosis of thoracic spine.

Labs
Fibrillin gene mutation identified on molecular studies.

Imaging
CXR/CT/MR: marked dilatation of ascending aorta. XR, plain: thoracic and lumbar kyphoscoliosis. Echo: **mitral valve prolapse.**

Micro Pathology
Cystic medial necrosis of aorta may lead to **dissection, rupture, aneurysm,** or **aortic insufficiency**; elastic lung fibers tortuous and thickened; emphysema formation.

Treatment
Spine bracing; ophthalmologic correction; endocarditis prophylaxis; beta-blockers to slow enlargement of aortic root; annual echocardiograms to evaluate aortic root diameter; composite valve graft replacement of aortic root when diameter exceeds 55 mm; aortic valve replacement.

Discussion
A systemic connective tissue disease characterized by an **autosomal-dominant** pattern of inheritance, Marfan's syndrome is due to a defective chromosome 15 **fibrillin gene**, a glycoprotein secreted by fibroblasts that acts as a scaffolding for the deposition of elastin.

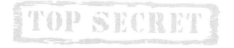

ANSWER KEY

1. Adult Respiratory Distress Syndrome (ARDS)
2. Asbestosis
3. Asthma
4. Atelectasis—Postoperative
5. Bronchiectasis
6. Churg–Strauss Syndrome
7. COPD—Chronic Bronchitis
8. COPD—Emphysema
9. Carbon Dioxide Narcosis
10. Fat Embolism
11. Hypersensitivity Pneumonitis
12. Idiopathic Pulmonary Fibrosis (IPF)
13. Lung Carcinoma
14. Malignant Mesothelioma
15. Pleural Effusion
16. Pneumothorax—Spontaneous
17. Pneumothorax—Tension
18. Primary Pulmonary Hypertension
19. Pulmonary Embolism
20. Sarcoidosis
21. Silicosis
22. Breast—Cystosarcoma Phyllodes
23. Breast—Fat Necrosis
24. Breast—Fibrocystic Disease
25. Breast—Inflammatory Carcinoma
26. Breast—Intraductal Papilloma
27. Breast—Lobular Carcinoma
28. Breast—Paget's Disease
29. Breast Carcinoma
30. Breast Fibroadenoma
31. Cervical Carcinoma (In Situ)
32. Choriocarcinoma
33. Desmoid Tumor
34. Dysmenorrhea
35. Endometrial Carcinoma
36. Endometriosis
37. Hydatidiform Mole
38. Menopause
39. Ovarian Cancer
40. Ovarian Cyst—Follicular
41. Ovarian Teratoma
42. Polycystic Ovarian Syndrome
43. Primary Amenorrhea—Turner's Syndrome
44. Uterine Fibroids
45. Uterine Leiomyosarcoma
46. Vulvar Carcinoma
47. Vulvar Leukoplakia
48. Vulvar Malignant Melanoma
49. Ectopic Pregnancy
50. Postpartum Hemorrhage
51. Postpartum Thrombophlebitis
52. Sheehan's Syndrome
53. Toxemia of Pregnancy—Preeclampsia
54. Acute Angle-Closure Glaucoma
55. Benign Positional Vertigo
56. Cribriform Plate Fracture
57. Deafness—Sensorineural
58. Labyrinthitis
59. Obstructive Sleep Apnea
60. Open-Angle Glaucoma
61. Presbycusis
62. Presbyopia
63. Pseudotumor Cerebri
64. Retinitis Pigmentosa
65. Retinoblastoma
66. Uveitis
67. Acute Lymphocytic Leukemia (ALL)
68. Acute Myelogenous Leukemia (AML)
69. Anemia—Aplastic
70. Anemia—Autoimmune Hemolytic
71. Antiphospholipid Antibody Syndrome
72. Burkitt's Lymphoma
73. Chronic Lymphocytic Leukemia (CLL)
74. Chronic Myelogenous Leukemia (CML)
75. Deep Venous Thrombosis
76. Disseminated Intravascular Coagulation (DIC)
77. Dysbetalipoproteinemia
78. Hairy Cell Leukemia
79. Henoch–Schönlein Purpura
80. Histiocytosis X—Eosinophilic Granuloma
81. Histiocytosis X—Hand–Schüller–Christian Disease
82. Histiocytosis X—Letterer–Siwe Disease
83. Hodgkin's Lymphoma
84. Idiopathic Thrombocytopenic Purpura (ITP)

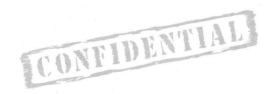

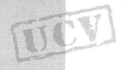

QUESTIONS

1. Your 65-year-old patient has hypertension. He presented to the emergency room yesterday saying that he heard a "click" in his head, and then suddenly experienced sharp neck pain. You suspect that a developmental berry aneurysm has ruptured in:

    A: The arterioles in kidney, bowel, or liver
    B: An artery in the circle of Willis
    C: The ascending portion of the arch of the aorta
    D: The middle meningeal artery
    E: The retina

2. What hormone is responsible for insulin resistance in gestational diabetes mellitus?

    A: hCG
    B: hPL
    C: Estrogen
    D: LH
    E: Progesterone

3. It's 3 AM in the busy ER on the first really cold night of the year where you are moonlighting for some extra money. A 17-year-old comes in complaining of shortness of breath. He states he was just in his new apartment all night watching TV. He became acutely short of breath and called 911. On physical exam he is breathing at a rate of 30 but has a normal lung exam and appears an odd pink color, so you put a finger oxygen sat meter on him and it quickly reads 100%, an ECG is normal. He appears in severe respiratory distress. You perform a diagnostic test, which reveals the correct and best diagnosis below.

    A: Asbestos exposure
    B: Asthma exacerbation
    C: Carbon monoxide poisoning
    D: Pneumonia
    E: Pulmonary embolism

4. An 18-year-old female presents to your office in respiratory distress after taking a couple of aspirins for a headache. After further questioning, you discover she also has a history of asthma and nasal polyps. Why did aspirin ingestion by this patient resulted in respiratory distress?

    A: Leukotrienes production
    B: Phospholipase A2 deficiency
    C: Prostacyclins production
    D: Prostaglandins production
    E: Thromboxane production

5. A patient comes to see you because he has been weak and falling down a lot. During the interview you note that he is suspicious and irritable. On

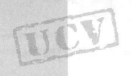

physical exam, you note that his skin is pale, his tarsal plates are also pale and a loss of vibration sense over the legs and trunk. His legs show a symmetric weakness with decreased deep tendon reflexes. The leading theory for the pathophysiology of this disorder relates to which of the following:

A: Anamolous insertion of even chain fatty acids into membrane lipids
B: Anomalous insertion of odd chain fatty acids into membrane lipids
C: Increased vitamin A intake.
D: Lack of methylmalonyl CoA.
E: Lack of propionyl CoA.

6. A 25-year-old woman with regular menses is given an estrogen challenge. The challenge consists of exogenous estrogen supplementation to see if LH hormone would increase. When would this be most effective?

A: Estradiol 20 days after menses
B: Estrogen 10 days after menses
C: Progesterone 10 days after onset of menses
D: Progesterone 20 days after the onset of menses
E: Synthetic FSH 15 days after the onset of menses

7. A 10-year-old female presents to the pediatric emergency room after excessive bleeding from a cut on her face. During the history you ascertain that she has been to the emergency room five times before with bleeding problems. You also find out that her mother has von Willebrand's disease. The patient's quantitative assay for factor VIII is shown to be reduced. What other lab abnormalities would you expect?

A: Increased PTT; normal platelet count, bleeding time and PT
B: Increased bleeding time; decreased platelet count; normal PT and PTT
C: Increased bleeding time and PTT; normal PT and platelet count
D: Increased bleeding time; normal platelet count, PT, PTT
E: Increased bleeding time, PT, PTT; decreased platelet count

8. Your patient presents with symptoms of fatigue, and shortness of breath. She claims that her symptoms have been getting progressively worse over the last couple of months. You notice that she looks a little pale to you. You take a blood test. The laboratory sends back a result that says that this patient's red blood cells are microcytic and hypochromic, there is decreased serum iron and decreased total iron-binding capacity. Your possible diagnosis is:

A: Anemia of chronic disease
B: β thalassemia minor
C: Folate deficiency anemia
D: Iron deficiency anemia
E: Pernicious anemia

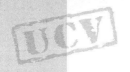

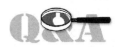

9. Your patient presents with a 25-year pack history of smoking. Recently, he has been experiencing shortness of breath and some sputum production. You order pulmonary function tests. What does functional vital capacity represent?

   A: Everything but residual volume
   B: Inspiratory capacity and functional reserve capacity
   C: Tidal volume, expiratory reserve volume, residual volume
   D: Tidal volume and inspiratory reserve volume
   E: Total lung capacity minus inspiratory reserve volume

10. A 25-year-old female presents to her obstetrician because she wants to make sure that it is all right for her to become pregnant. History reveals that she fainted once while jogging 2 weeks ago. She also reports lightheadedness and shortness of breath with only a small amount of exertion. The patient also reports that she fatigues easily and is concerned. The patient denies tobacco, alcohol, and recreational drugs. Both of her parents are in their 60s and healthy. The patient's pulse is 76 and her blood pressure is 118/75. Physical exam is remarkable for a crescendo-decrescendo systolic ejection murmur. It is auscultated best to the right of the sternum and radiates to her neck. Which of the following murmurs does this patient most likely have?

    A: Aortic insufficiency
    B: Aortic stenosis
    C: Mitral insufficiency
    D: Mitral prolapse
    E: Mitral stenosis

11. A 38-year-old female has just been diagnosed with breast cancer. She has since read a variety of books, journals, and newspaper articles on the topic. She comes to see you in your office today. She asks you which of the following signs of breast cancer affect prognosis. Choose the best answer.

    A: Size of the tumor
    B: Number of involved lymph nodes
    C: Presence or absence of estrogen and progesterone receptors
    D: Degree of new vessel growth that is feeding the tumor
    E: All of the above

12. A 50-year-old man consults you for his severe headaches. He describes his headaches as lasting about 2 hours, severe, burning, nonthrobbing and always located over his left eye. Each night they tend to wake him up for several weeks in a row, then he doesn't have them again for several months. He's had these headaches for about 5 years. He denies any history of headaches in his family. What type of headache does he have?

    A: Classic migraine
    B: Cluster headache

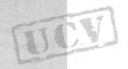

C: Common migraine
D: Intracranial bleed
E: Tension headache

13. A 30-year-old female and her 32-year-old husband are trying to conceive a child. They present to your office asking when should they have intercourse to maximize their chance of becoming pregnant. Assuming that both are in good reproductive health and that the woman has a 28-day menstrual cycle, what is the best answer?

   A: Intercourse on day 2
   B: Intercourse on day 5
   C: Intercourse on day 10
   D: Intercourse on day 13
   E: Intercourse on day 28

14. A child was recently diagnosed with L1 leukemia. This is your first meeting with the parents and child after the diagnosis. They ask you if there is a genetic basis for the disease. You respond that it is associated with which translocation?

   A: t(4;11)
   B: t(6;12)
   C: t(8;14)
   D: t(8;21)
   E: t(15;17)

15. A 2-year-old toddler is brought into the emergency room by his parents with dyspnea, diaphoresis, and wheezing (inspiratory and expiratory). The patient has a history of severe asthma for which he has been on inhaled corticosteriod and albuterol for some time. The parents have given the child several doses of the albuterol with no improvement. The child was alone in a room playing with his toys when the parents found him in distraught. The child is unable to vocalize any sounds. Which of the following is the best option to explain the child's current status?

   A: The child is suffering from an acute asthmatic attack.
   B: The child has aspirated something likely found on the floor and it is partially obstructing his airway passage.
   C: The parents are mis-administering the albuterol.
   D: The child has an inherent inability to speak.
   E: The child is having a panic attack.

16. A 26-year-old African American woman comes to the her doctor complaining of "spotting" when she is not on her period, severe pain with "a lot of blood loss" during her periods and abdominal pain. She has had these complaints for several years but never came to see a doctor for it until today. She is sexually active but denies having intercourse since her last menstrual

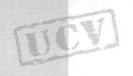
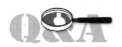

period 3 weeks ago. She does not think she is pregnant. Her urine and blood B-HCG levels are in the normal range for a non-pregnant female. On pelvic exam, her uterus feels enlarged and is about the size of an 8-week uterus. Which of the following best explains what we see with this patient?

A: The patient suffers from pseudopshyesis.
B: The patient suffers from uterine fibroids.
C: The patient has uterine cancer.
D: She is pregnant with a negative B-HCG.
E: She is 8 weeks pregnant.

17. A 76-year-old male with a 20-pack year history of smoking comes to the physician complaining of shortness of breath. The patient is also complaining of increased sputum production. Physicial exam reveals increased anterior-posterior diameter of the chest. The physician requested spirometry data and advised the patient to stop smoking. What do you expect to see on spirometry data?

A: Decreased total lung capacity.
B: Increased inspiratory capacity.
C: Inspiratory reverse volume will be increased.
D: Tital volume will be increased.
E: The volume of total lung capacity minus vital capacity will be increased.

18. A 58-year-old former alcoholic is brought in by his wife to see you in clinic. She tells you in private that she's worried her husband is back to drinking because his face "is red all the time these days." When you speak with the patient, he denies any alcohol use in the last 12 years. He says his only problems are that he's been "wheezing a lot lately" and that his "stomach's been acting up—lots of diarrhea." The physical exam is normal and vitals are within normal ranges. Routine screening reveals no serum ethanol. However, his liver function tests return abnormal results. Which of these tests would be the next appropriate diagnostic exam?

A: Barium swallow test
B: Colonoscopy
C: Echocardiogram
D: Liver biopsy
E: Urine metabolite analysis

19. A 4-year-old patient who is adopted is suspected of having hemophilia A. Laboratory tests that would confirm the diagnosis include:

A: Increased PTT, normal PT, normal bleeding time
B: Increased PTT, increased PT, increased fibrin split products
C: Increased bleeding time, normal PT, normal PTT, abnormal risto-cetin assay

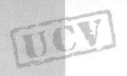

D: Normal PT, increased PTT, increased INR

E: Increased PTT, normal PT, increased INR

20. Estrogen is important for many different actions in the body, including the LH surge, growth of the follicle, and myometrial excitability. Which of the following is another function of estrogen?

A: Endometrial proliferation

B: Increased body temperature around ovulation

C: Production of thick cervical mucous

D: Spiral artery development in the endometrium

E: Uterine smooth muscle relaxation

ANSWERS

A: The arterioles in kidney, bowel, or liver [Incorrect] Aneurysms at these sites are common in polyarteritis nodosa.

B: An artery in the circle of Willis [Correct] This is frequent place for developmental berry aneurysms that may rupture and cause subarachnoid bleeds, especially if the patient is hypertensive.

C: The ascending portion of the arch of the aorta [Incorrect] tertiary syphilis commonly causes an aneurysm here.

D: The middle meningeal artery [Incorrect] Rupture of middle meningeal artery is commonly associated with an extradural hematoma caused by trauma. The patient would, characteristically, experience a hit to the head, not feel any symptoms, and then suddenly lapse into a coma due to ischemia in the brain caused by increased pressure of the hematoma.

E: The retina [Incorrect] This is a frequent place for diabetic microaneurysms.

2. B

A: hCG [Incorrect] hCG is not believed to play a role in development of GDM.

B: hPL [Correct] Human placental lactogen is believed to be the main culprit in the development of GDM in pregnant women. HPL is produced in the placenta and is important for ensuring a constant nutrient supply to the fetus. HPL causes lipolysis and hence an increase in free fatty acids. It also has diabetogenic effects on the mother and leads to increased levels of insulin and development of diabetes.

C: Estrogen [Incorrect] Estrogen is not believed to play a role in development of GDM.

D: LH [Incorrect] Luteinizing hormone is not believed to play a role in development of GDM.

E: Progesterone [Incorrect] Progesterone is not believed to play a role in development of GDM.

3. C

A: Asbestos exposure [Incorrect] Typically in shipyard workers from years ago. This disease process is not normally acute and leads to the classic cancer mesothelioma.

B: Asthma exacerbation [Incorrect] You would expect to see a lower oxygen sat along with wheezing or decreased air movement on exam.

C: Carbon monoxide poisoning [Correct] Anyone who comes in with a sat of 100% and in severe respiratory distress with a normal exam should be considered for CO poisoning. This can happen from car exhaust or an old gas heater which has just been started up on a cold night. The diagnostic test is the ABG which reveals carboxyhemoglobin. The treatement is oxygen, hyperbaric if avail. Carbon

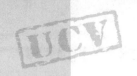

monoxide has a much higher affinity for hemoglobin and once it binds it causes the other 3 sites in the hemoglobin to be less likely to bind oxygen.

D: Pneumonia [Incorrect] This again could be a possibility but less likely if the patient is in this much distress and has a 100% oxygen sat.

E: Pulmonary embolism [Incorrect] Again, the sat is too high, although the acute onset of the illness is in line with this diagnosis. A blood gas would be useful in this setting where you would expect a low Pao_2.

4. A

A: Leukotrienes production [Correct] Aspirin like NSAIDs and acetaminophen blocks COX-1 and COX-2 enzymes in the arachidonic acid metabolism. However, lipoxygenase enzyme pathway is not blocked, thus funneling most of arachidonic acid through the lipoxygenase pathway that produces Leukotrienes (LTB, LTC, LTD). LTs are responsible for increased bronchial tone, i.e., bronchospasm, causing respiratory distress symptoms in this patient.

B: Phospholipase A2 deficiency [Incorrect] Deficiency in phospholipase A2 would mean that no arachidonic acid is produced. If there is deficiency in arachidonic acid, than aspirin has no negative effect in that situation and would not cause respiratory distress.

C: Prostacyclins production [Incorrect] Prostacyclins are by-products of acrochidonic acid metabolism via COX enzyme pathway. Since aspirin blocks both COX-1 and COX-2, no PGIs will be produced. In addition, PGIs are responsible for decreased bronchial and vascular tones, and decreased platelet aggregation.

D: Prostaglandins production [Incorrect] Prostaglandins are by products of acrochidonic acid metabolism via COX enzyme pathway. Since aspirin blocks both COX-1 and COX-2, no PGE/PGF will be produced. Prostaglandins are responsible for decreased bronchial and vascular tones.

E: Thromboxane production [Incorrect] Thromboxane is a by-product of acrochidonic acid metabolism via COX enzyme pathway. Since aspirin blocks both COX-1 and COX-2, no TXA will be produced. TXA, however, can increase bronchial tone and result in bronchospasm leading to respiratory distress.

5. B

A: Anamolous insertion of even chain fatty acids into membrane lipids [Incorrect] Even if you have no idea of the answer, that there are two opposite answers suggest that one of them is the correct answer

B: Anomalous insertion of odd chain fatty acids into membrane lipids [Correct] The patient is pale which might suggest anemia. The most

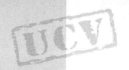
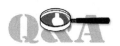

consistent sign of B_{12} deficiency is loss of vibration sense in the legs which can extend to the trunk. Changes in mental status are frequent. These changes include irritability, confusion, suspiciousness, and emotional instability. Lack of cobalamin leads to accumulation of methylmalonyl CoA and proprionyl CoA. Excess propionyl CoA leads to displacement of succinlyl CoA, which results in formation of anamolous odd chain fatty acids in membrane lipids.

C: Increased vitamin A intake. [Incorrect] This is a distractor and also a hint that this question is about vitamins. Always use the answers to help guide your thinking when you don't know the answer to the question.

D: Lack of methylmalonyl CoA. [Incorrect] Methylmalonyl CoA will be increased with vitamin B_{12} deficiency.

E: Lack of propionyl CoA. [Incorrect] Propionyl CoA will be increased with vitamin B_{12} deficiency.

6.   B

A: Estradiol 20 days after menses [Incorrect] If estrodiol was given 20 days after menses then the cycle would already be in the luteal phase. Once in the luteal phase, LH will not rise until the next cycle.

B: Estrogen 10 days after menses [Correct] High levels of estrogen are needed to stimulate adequate LH production.

C: Progesterone 10 days after onset of menses [Incorrect] Progesterone typically very low during the follicular phase. It does not stimulate LH.

D: Progesterone 20 days after the onset of menses [Incorrect] Progesterone does not stimulate LH.

E: Synthetic FSH 15 days after the onset of menses [Incorrect] FSH is not the principal stimulator of LH.

7.   C

A: Increased PTT; normal platelet count, bleeding time and PT [Incorrect] These lab abnormalities would be expected with either hemophilia A (factor VIII deficiency) or hemophilia B (factor IX deficiency), not von Willebrand's disease.

B: Increased bleeding time; decreased platelet count; normal PT and PTT [Incorrect] These lab abnormalities would be expected in patients with thrombocytopenia, not von Willebrand's disease.

C: Increased bleeding time and PTT; normal PT and platelet count [Correct] Increased bleeding time and increased PTT would be expected in von Willebrand's disease, which from the history and physical is this patient's most likely diagnosis. von Willebrand's disease is usually an autosomal dominant condition.

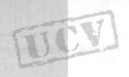

D: Increased bleeding time; normal platelet count, PT, PTT [Incorrect] Increased bleeding time only would be seen in patients with either vascular bleeding or possibly with platelet defects.

E: Increased bleeding time, PT, PTT; decreased platelet count [Incorrect] Increased bleeding time, PT, and PTT with decreased platelet count would be expected in patients with disseminated intravascular coagulation. A patient with DIC would have a much more acute presentation.

8.   A

A: Anemia of chronic disease [Correct] Anemia of chronic disease may present as macrocytic, normocytic, or microcytic. The key to answering this question is remembering the lab abnormalities for this disease: low iron and low TIBC. This type of anemia may be associated with chronic inflammatory states such as rheumatoid arthritis.

B: β thalassemia minor [Incorrect] Thalassemia would present clinically as microcytic and hypochromic, but levels of hemoglobin A2 would be markedly increased.

C: Folate deficiency anemia [Incorrect] Folate deficiency anemia presents as macrocytic, not microcytic.

D: Iron deficiency anemia [Incorrect] The lab abnormalities for iron deficiency anemia would be decreased iron, but increased TIBC.

E: Pernicious anemia [Incorrect] Pernicious anemia is caused by a deficiency of vitamin B_{12} and manifests as macrocytic, not microcytic. Vitamin B_{12} deficiency is also associated with neurological abnormalities, as opposed to folate deficiency anemia.

9.   A

A: Everything but residual volume [Correct] Vital capacity is the maximum inspiratory and expiratory function that a lung can perform. VC includes every parameter such as ERV, IRV, TV, except RV which is a fixed volume of air in lung after maximum expiration.

B: Inspiratory capacity and functional reserve capacity [Incorrect] FVC includes ERV, IRV, TV, except RV.

C: Tidal volume, expiratory reserve volume, residual volume [Incorrect] FVC includes ERV, IRV, TV, except RV.

D: Tidal volume and inspiratory reserve volume [Incorrect] FVC includes ERV, IRV, TV, except RV.

E: Total lung capacity minus inspiratory reserve volume [Incorrect] FVC includes ERV, IRV, TV, except RV.

10.   B

A: Aortic insufficiency [Incorrect] The murmur of aortic insufficiency is that of a high-pitched "blowing" diastolic murmur. It is usually

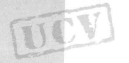
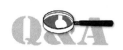

auscultated best at the left sternal border. These patients often have a widened pulse pressure as well.

B: Aortic stenosis [Correct] The presentation above is typical for aortic stenosis. This may be secondary to a congenital bicuspid aortic valve. The murmur is a crescendo-decrescendo systolic ejection murmur.

C: Mitral insufficiency [Incorrect] Mitral insufficiency typically has a high pitched decrescendo holosystolic murmur.

D: Mitral prolapse [Incorrect] The murmur of mitral valve prolapse is systolic with a midsystolic click.

E: Mitral stenosis [Incorrect] Mitral stenosis presents with a rumbling late diastolic murmur which follows the opening snap of the valve.

11.   E

A: Size of the tumor [Incorrect] The smaller the size of the primary tumor the better the outcome.

B: Number of involved lymph nodes [Incorrect] The fewer lymph nodes that are involved the better the prognosis.

C: Presence or absence of estrogen and progesterone receptors [Incorrect] The presence of these receptors indicates a more differentiated type of breast cancer and is useful in drug therapy (e.g., Tamoxifen use)

D: Degree of new vessel growth that is feeding the tumor [Incorrect] The greater the vessels that supply the cancer, the greater is the chance of metastasis.

E: All of the above [Correct] See above for individual explanations.

12.   B

A: Classic migraine. [Incorrect] A classic migraine is usually a unilateral throbbing headache, associated with an aura, scintillating scotomas, photophobia, phonophobia, nausea, and vomiting.

B: Cluster headache. [Correct] This is a typical description of a cluster headache, which mainly occur in men, are located around one eye, occur at the same time of day for a period of time ("clustered" in time) with periods of weeks or months with no headaches.

C: Common migraine. [Incorrect] A common migraine is often bilateral and periorbital without the classic aura of a classic migraine.

D: Intracranial bleed. [Incorrect] An intracranial bleed is usually described as "the worst headache of my life," occurs acutely, not chronically as the headache in this case.

E: Tension headache. [Incorrect] A tension headache is usually bilateral, non-throbbing occipital pain that is often described as a tight band around the head.

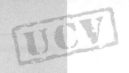

13. D

    A: Intercourse on day 2 [Incorrect] This is the menstrual phase and no ovum is present for fertilization to occur.

    B: Intercourse on day 5 [Incorrect] This is the follicular phase and no ovum has yet been released for fertilization.

    C: Intercourse on day 10 [Incorrect] This is the follicular phase and no ovum has yet been released for fertilization.

    D: Intercourse on day 13 [Correct] Ideally the woman will ovulate on day 14 of her cycle. Once her egg is released it will be viable for 24 hours. The couple can maximize their chance of pregnancy by having intercourse within 24 hours before and after the time at which the ovum is released—which is on day 14.

    E: Intercourse on day 28 [Incorrect] This is the menstrual phase and no ovum is present for fertilization to occur.

14. A

    A: t(4;11) [Correct] t(4;11) is associated with L1.

    B: t(6;12) [Incorrect] t(6;12) is associated with M1, 2, and 4.

    C: t(8;14) [Incorrect] t(8;14) is associated with Burkitt's lymphoma

    D: t(8;21) [Incorrect] t(8;21) is associated with M2.

    E: t(15;17) [Incorrect] t(15;17) is associated with M3.

15. B

    A: The child is suffering from an acute asthmatic attack. [Incorrect] This is possible but unlikely given that the patient has both inspiratory and expiratory wheezing, has had no improvement with multiple doses of his albuterol, and is unable to vocalize at all.

    B: The child has aspirated something likely found on the floor and it is partially obstructing his airway passage. [Correct] This is the likely answer given that the patient is wheezing at all times, has had no improvement with albuterol, and is unable to vocalize at all. Toddlers place many things in their mouths that can cause them to have such a dangerous clinical picture. Remember, all that wheezes is not asthma.

    C: The parents are mis-administering the albuterol. [Incorrect] This is a possibility but is unlikely if the parents have been using the albuterol with their child for some time. There is no mention in the question that the parents recently started using inhalers with their child.

    D: The child has an inherent inability to speak. [Incorrect]. This does not explain any of the other findings.

    E: The child is having a panic attack. [Incorrect] Children at this age do not have panic attacks. Panic attacks begin in teenage years or the second decade of life.

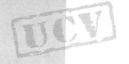
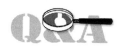

16. B

   A: The patient suffers from pseudopshyesis. [Incorrect] Pseudopshyesis is a complex psychological condition where the patient thinks she is pregnant and but is not. Such patients will often "look" pregnant.

   B: The patient suffers from uterine fibroids. [Correct] African American women have a higher incidence of getting uterine fibroids. This patient has the classical presentation of someone who has uterine fibroids—abnormal uterine spotting, dysmenorrhea, and menorhagia.

   C: The patient has uterine cancer. [Incorrect] Such a definitive statement cannot be made without further workup, including histological tissue for analysis. Statistically she is too young to have developed uterine cancer. Her symptoms do not resemble uterine cancer.

   D: She is pregnant with a negative B-HCG. [Incorrect] The patient is not pregnant if both her urine B-HCG and blood B-HCG are negative.

   E: She is 8 weeks pregnant. [Incorrect] The patient is not pregnant if both her urine B-HCG and blood B-HCG are negative. Her uterus is enlarged to an 8 week size because of her large fibroids.

17. E

   A: Decreased total lung capacity. [Incorrect] In COPD patients have an increase in TLC.

   B: Increased inspiratory capacity. [Incorrrect] In COPD this value is probably slightly decreased considering the lungs are already hyperinflated.

   C: Inspiratory reverse volume will be increased. [Incorrect] This value will also most likely be decreased given the lung hyperinflated state.

   D: Tital volume will be increased. [Incorrect] This most probably will be decreased considering the lung is already hyperinflated.

   E: The volume of total lung capacity minus vital capacity will be increased. [Correct] This TLC-VC represents the residual volume. An increase of residual volume is the hallmark of COPD.

18. E

   A: Barium swallow test [Incorrect] This test is not indicated. The patient is not complaining of difficulties with swallowing or presenting with heartburn/reflux.

   B: Colonoscopy [Incorrect] This is an invasive procedure and is typically performed in the setting of heightened suspicion for colorectal cancer (e.g., after a guaiac test, consistent history, etc.).

   C: Echocardiogram [Incorrect] There is no indication for an echocardiogram at this point. Carcinoid syndrome is associated with heart findings in up to 50% of patients, causing plaque-like, fibrous endocardial thickening that classically involves the right side of the heart

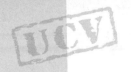

and often causes retraction and fixation of the leaflets of the tricuspid and pulmonary valves. However, it is premature to obtain an echocardiogram before the diagnosis has been established.

D: Liver biopsy [Incorrect] This is an invasive procedure and should only be performed if tissue is required. Abnormal liver function tests can resolve transiently and are not an immediate indication for biopsy.

E: Urine metabolite analysis [Correct] The patient's presentation (flushing, wheezing, diarrhea) and abnormal LFTs are suspicious for a carcinoid tumor that has metastasized from the small intestine to the liver and/or beyond. Carcinoids are potentially malignant tumors of enterochromaffin/Kulchitsky cell origin. They typically elaborate serotonin, which causes many of the effects of carcinoid syndrome. The serotonin is subsequently metabolized by monoamine oxidase to 5-hydroxyindoleacetic acid (5-HIAA) and is excreted in the urine. 5-HIAA in a 24-hour urine collection verifies the diagnosis of carcinoid syndrome and can be used in subsequent follow-up of carcinoids.

19.   A

A: Increased PTT, normal PT, normal bleeding time [Correct] This profile is compatible with the factor VIII deficiency of hemophilia A.

B: Increased PTT, increased PT, increased fibrin split products. [Incorrect] This profile is compatible with DIC.

C: Increased bleeding time, normal PT, normal PTT, abnormal ristocetin assay [Incorrect] This profile is consistent with von Willibrand's disease.

D: Normal PT, Increased PTT, increased INR [Incorrect] This profile is consistent with warfarin therapy.

E: Increased PTT, normal PT, increased INR [Incorrect] This profile is consistent with heparin therapy.

20.   A

A: Endometrial proliferation [Correct] Estrogen is responsible for endometrial proliferation.

B: Increased body temperature around ovulation [Incorrect] Progesterone is responsible for increased body temperature around ovulation.

C: Production of thick cervical mucous [Incorrect] Progesterone is responsible for the production of thick cervical mucous.

D: Spiral artery development in the endometrium [Incorrect] Progesterone is responsible for spiral artery development in the endometrium.

E: Uterine smooth muscle relaxation [Incorrect] Progesterone is responsible for uterine smooth muscle relaxation.